CHOICE
Psychology

FREEMON, Frank R. Sleep research; a critical review. C. C. Thomas, 1972. 205p il tab bibl 72-75915. 14.50. ISBN 0-398-02540-1

An excellent book: exhaustive, yet concise presentation and explanation of sleep as a phenomenon and the current state of research make it invaluable as a reference work as well as a source book. Freemon's authority is well established by abundant research and publication. The scope of contents is exceptionally wide, encompassing all aspects of sleep and sleep research — physiology (normal and pathological), types of sleep (REM and non-REM), comparative sleep studies (animal and human), dream processes, sleep deprivation, drug-influence, arousal, and an outstanding, eclectic chapter on the theories of sleep from mythological-symbolic explanations to the most modern clinical and nonclinical theories. Impressive, all-inclusive bibliography, clear illustrations and graphs (EEG, etc.), excellent index. All college and public libraries should have this book, supplementing and complementing valuable basic works and research publications such as W. C. Dement's "Eye movements during sleep" in *The oculomotor system,* ed. by M. B. Bender (1964) and "The biological role of 'REM sleep" in *Sleep: physiology and pathology,* ed. by A. Kales ; *Physiological correlates of dreaming* ed. by C. D. Clemente ; and "Some impli-

CHOICE   *SEPT. '73*

Psychology

FREEMON

cations of sleep research for psychiatry," by I. Feinberg and E. V. Evarts in *Neurobiological aspects of psychopathology,* ed. by J. Zubin and C. Shagass (1969). Highly recommended to undergraduate as well as graduate students in the fields of medicine, physiology, psychology, and anthropology.

Sleep Research

A Critical Review

By

FRANK R. FREEMON, M.D.

Assistant Professor
Department of Neurology
Vanderbilt University School of Medicine
Nashville, Tennessee

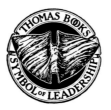

CHARLES C THOMAS • PUBLISHER
Springfield • Illinois • U.S.A.

Published and Distributed Throughout the World by
CHARLES C THOMAS • PUBLISHER
BANNERSTONE HOUSE
301-327 East Lawrence Avenue, Springfield, Illinois, U.S.A.

© 1972, by CHARLES C THOMAS • PUBLISHER
ISBN 0-398-02540-1
Library of Congress Catalog Card Number: 72-75915

With THOMAS BOOKS *careful attention is given to all details of
manufacturing and design. It is the Publisher's desire to present books
that are satisfactory as to their physical qualities and artistic possibilities
and appropriate for their particular use.* THOMAS BOOKS *will be true
to those laws of quality that assure a good name and good will.*

Printed in the United States of America
PP-22

To my wife,

Linda Mary Freemon nee Jones

PREFACE

SCIENTISTS from many disciplines have been drawn to the study of the surprisingly complex behavior of sleep. Psychologists, physiologists, psychoanalysts, biochemists, and clinicians have approached sleep research from different backgrounds. The field is fragmented, the literature scattered, the nomenclature confusing, the underlying concepts complex. This book attempts to review this field for the nonspecialist.

There are many books on sleep. The past decade has seen the publication of volumes on sleep written or edited by Bertini (1970), Clemente (1967), Foulkes (1966), Gastaut, Lugaresi, Berti Ceroni, and Coccagna (1968), Hartmann (1967b, 1970), Jones (1970), Jouvet (1965), Kales (1969), Kety, Evarts, and Williams (1967), Kleitman (1963), Koella (1967), Kramer (1969), Luce and Segal (1966), Madow and Snow (1970), Magoun (1963), Murray (1965), Oswald (1962), Petre-Quadens (1972), Ullman and Montague (1970), Webb (1968), Williams and Webb (1966), Witkin and Lewis (1967), and others. The present book is not intended to serve as the straw which collapses the sleep wing of the library, but to supplement these other volumes as a critical review of or introduction to sleep research.

In order to keep this volume short, some aspects of sleep research have been disregarded. Sleep-related phenomena not covered include hibernation (the reader is referred to the monograph by Mrosovsky, 1971) and electrosleep (see Wulfsohn and Sances, 1970, or Wageneder and Schuy, 1970). This book, also for sake of brevity, fails to consider certain minority viewpoints. For example, some authorities still consider narcolepsy to be a form of epilepsy (Elliot, 1971). Refutation of this relationship would take a paragraph; I think that this concept is so inherently unlikely that it does not rate a paragraph. The sleep literature is so massive that only the most recent articles are quoted.

I hope this short monograph will be of value to the life scientist, clinician, or advanced student who desires an introduction to the interesting, important, yet sometimes exasperating field of sleep research.

FRANK R. FREEMON

ACKNOWLEDGMENTS

THE author thanks the many scientists, some close colleagues, and others he has never met, who have read and criticized portions of this book. Acknowledgment is due the typists of the manuscript, Lita Twells and Sandy Scholler, the bibliographic assistance provided by the monthly *Sleep Bulletin* of the UCLA Brain Information Service, and the United States government which has supported most of the research reviewed in this volume including the author's (US Air Force grant AFOSR-62-13 to RL Williams, National Aeronautics and Space Administration contract NSR 05-007-158 to WR Adey, and Public Health Service special fellowship 1 F11 NB 2050 NSRB). The author's wife provided most of the literary quotations in the book.

The following are reproduced with the permission of the copyright holders. Figure 2 is a copy of an original work in the Art Institute of Chicago. Figures 3, 6, 7, 8, and 13 are from *Experimental Neurology* (Academic Press); Figures 9, 11, 12, and 14 are from *Comprehensive Psychiatry* (Grune and Stratton), and Figure 5 is from *Electroencephalography and Clinical Neurophysiology* (Elsevier). Quotations from articles by P. Solomon and S.A.K. Wilson are reproduced with the permission of the editors of the *New England Journal of Medicine* and *Brain* respectively. Excerpts are reproduced with permission from Senator A.V. Watkins' *Enough Rope* (Prentice-Hall), from Eric Ambler's *Epitaph for a Spy* (Knopf), from J.E. Pfeiffer's *Emergence of Man* (Harper and Row), from S.L.A. Marshall's *Night Drop* (Little, Brown), from Bruce Catton's *A Stillness at Appomattox* (Doubleday and Company), and from Arthur Koestler's *Darkness at Noon* (Macmillan). Author and publisher have granted permission to reproduce excerpts from Dement and Wolpert's article in the *Journal of Experimental Psychology*, 1958, from Foulkes article in the *Journal of Abnormal Psychology*, 1962 (American Psychological Association), from Dement's chapter in *The Oculomotor System* (Harper and Row), from Dement's article in *Experimental Neurology*, 1967 (Academic

Press), and from an editorial in the *Journal of Nervous and Mental Disease* (Williams and Wilkins). The author also thanks Drs. C.H. Markham, R.T. Pivik, and Olga Petre-Quadens for the privilege of reading prepublication copies of their forthcoming works.

F.R.F.

CONTENTS

Sleep Research

Chapter 1

NORMAL HUMAN SLEEP

There lay the gods and slept, Morpheus and Eclympasteyre, who was heir to the god of sleep, who slept and did none other toil. This cave was as dark everywhere about as the pit of hell. They had good leisure to snore in rivalry; who were the soundest sleeper! Some hung chin on breast and slept standing upright, their heads hidden; and some lay abed and slept the long days through.

This messenger came flying swiftly and cried, "Oh ho! Awake, and that anon!" It was in vain; none heard him. "Awake!" quoth he. "Who is it lies there?" And he blew his horn right in their ears and cried wondrous loud, "Awake!"

This god of sleep opened one eye and asked, "Who calls there?"

CHAUCER, *Book of the Duchess*

TWO SLEEP STATES

AN unequivocal definition of sleep evades us. The final scientific definition must be based on the sleeper's decreased ability to interact with his external environment. Subjective estimates of sleep latency, quality, and duration can compare the sleep of large populations, but the estimates become inaccurate as subject groups become smaller (Johns, 1971). In fact, as discussed more fully in the next chapter, a person lying quietly in bed may think he is awake when he is actually asleep. The recording of polygraphic variables throughout the night has provided a fuller description of sleep. The major discovery produced by all-night polygraphy is the existence of two separate types of sleep.

These two sleep states are defined by three separate polygraphic variables: electroencephalography, electromyography from the chin muscles, and eye movements. One sleep state, called nonrem sleep, contains slow waves, spindles, and K-complexes in the EEG record. No eye movements occur except for transient and slow eye movements as the sleeper first enters this stage. The electrical activity of the chin EMG decreases as one passes from wakefulness to nonrem sleep but

3

falls further, almost to zero, during the other type of sleep. This second type of sleep, called the rem state, has low voltage EEG activity mixed with bursts of theta waves and frequent conjugate eye movements. Although these two states are defined by these three polygraphic criteria, almost every variable measured shows differences between them. For example, penile erection occurs only during rem periods (Fisher et al., 1965; Karacan et al., 1965). Table I summarizes some of the many differences between these two states.

One of the most confusing aspects of sleep research is the shifting nomenclature of these two types of sleep. The original all-night sleep study of Dement and Kleitman (1957) classified sleep into four stages solely on the basis of the EEG. Stage 2 was characterized by spindles and K-complexes. Stage 3 contained more than 20 percent and stage 4 more than 50 percent of high voltage slow activity in the delta frequency band. Stage 1 occurred as the individual passed from wakefulness to sleep and also occurred later in the night associated with rapid eye movements. A confused terminology arose to separate these two types of stage 1. What is now called nonrem stage 1 was referred to as descending stage 1, 1 in quotation marks, sleep onset 1, drowsiness, transitional sleep, and several other terms. Rem sleep was termed ascending or emergent stage 1 or stage 1-REM. Many studies which failed to separate the two types of stage 1 are now worthless. For example, the average evoked response during "stage 1" given by Corletto et al. (1967) is a mixture of nonrem stage 1 and rem values in unknown proportion, and this study cannot be compared to other evoked response studies. Now we divide sleep into its two basic types, rem and nonrem, and further subdivide nonrem sleep into four numbered substages.

Many workers have suggested other names for rem and nonrem sleep. Some European scientists refer to rem as paradoxical sleep and usually call nonrem slow or spindle sleep. Scientists working with experimental animals frequently call the rem state deep sleep while many scientists working with human subjects refer to nonrem stages 3 and 4 as deep sleep. The concept of sleep depth turns out to be quite complicated and is discussed in Chapter 6. Some scientists working with the EEG refer to rem as desynchronized and nonrem as synchronized sleep. The term synchronization can mean different things. To some electroencephalographers such as Kooi (1971), waveforms

TABLE I

NONREM AND REM CHARACTERISTICS IN MAN

Measurement	Nonrem sleep	Rem Sleep	Reference
Scalp EEG	Slow waves and spindles	Low voltage, mixed frequency	Dement and Kleitman (1957)
Hippocampal EEG	Variable	Rhythmic theta activity	See Chapter 4
Eye movements	None or few slow movements	Conjugate rapid movements	Aserinsky and Kleitman (1955)
Chin EMG	Decreased from wakefulness	Almost absent	Berger (1961)
Body movements	A few gross movements	Twitches	Jacobson et al. (1964)
Respiration	Regular, deep	Variable, shallow	Snyder et al. (1964)
Heart rate	Regular, slow	Variable, rapid	Snyder et al. (1964)
Blood pressure	Below waking level	Variable	Williams and Cartwright (1969)
Penile erection	Absent	Present	Fisher et al. (1965)
Mentation	Thought-like, repetitive	Dream-like, dramatic	See Chapter 2
Galvanic skin response	Frequent	Rare	Broughton et al. (1965)

in different brain areas are said to be synchronized if they can be superimposed. Thus the alpha rhythm of relaxed wakefulness is synchronous over both hemispheres while the delta activity of nonrem sleep is asynchronous. In sleep research, however, slow rhythms are said to show synchronization, and fast activity is referred to as desynchronization. These terms are derived from a historical theory of the generation of EEG rhythms which postulated that cortical neurons firing together, that is, synchronously, would give slow waves while neurons firing independently or desynchronously would give fast activity. Even as it is used in sleep research this terminology breaks down. As one moves from wakefulness with a background rhythm of 8 to 12 cycles per second and enters nonrem sleep characterized by bursts of spindle waves at 12 to 15 cps, one is said to move from a desynchronized to synchronized state even though the background activity speeds up. Table II summarizes some of the many names for the rem and nonrem types of sleep.

In my opinion, the best terminology is the system suggested by Hartmann (1965). He refers to waking, nonrem sleep, and rem sleep

TABLE II

NOMENCLATURE OF SLEEP STATES

Rem	*Nonrem*	*Typical Reference*
paradoxical	orthodoxical	Jouvet (1960)
paradoxical	slow wave	Jouvet (1967)
para-sleep	ortho-sleep	Iwamura et al. (1967)
rhombencephalic	telencephalic	Jouvet (1961)
rhombencephalic	high voltage	Buendia et al. (1963)
rapid	slow	Allison (1965)
desynchronized	synchronized	Dunlop and Waks (1968)
LVF	HVS	Berger and Meier (1966)
low voltage fast	slow wave	Webb and Friedmann (1971)
D	S	Hartmann (1965)
A, D	B, C	Petre-Quadens (1966)
B	C, D, E	Davis et al. (1938)
S-A	S-1, S-2	Okuma and Akimoto (1966)
1	2, 3, 4	Dement and Kleitman (1957)
1	2	Goldie and Van Velzer (1965)
first sleep	second sleep	Roldan et al. (1963)
2	1	Prechtl (1965)
2	3, 4	Hoffman et al. (1955)
2	3, 4, 5, 6, 7	Toyoda (1964)
activated	ordinary	Dement (1958)
active	quiet	Parmalee et al. (1967)
restless	quiet	Cadilhac et al. (1961)
irregular	regular	Wolff (1959)
light	deep	Karacan et al. (1970)
deep	light	Carli and Zanchetti (1956)

by the capital letters W, S, and D. S might stand for synchronized, slow wave, spindle sleep while D might stand for desynchronized state or dreaming, depending upon one's physiological or psychological bias. Should future research describe other psychophysiological states of existence, say Zen meditation, these states could be incorporated into this system by selection of a descriptive letter, say Z. Though the W-S-D nomenclature is simple, descriptive, expandable, and without theoretical bias, it has not found general acceptance since its introduction. It is too late for new nomenclature. We are stuck with rem and norem, which will be used throughout this book. The conclusion is, when you describe a new phenomenon, try to devise a reasonable name for it right from the beginning.

The term *rem* is, of course, derived from the rapid eye movements of rem sleep. Some workers still use this term as an abbreviation for eye movements, such as referring to the periods of rem sleep between eye movements as "D state without REMs." In this book, however, rem sleep refers to a complete physiological state of which the eye movements are but one phenomenon. An enucleated animal will have no eye movements during sleep or wakefulness but will still have periods of rem sleep characterized by low voltage, mixed frequency EEG and markedly depressed chin EMG. Rem and nonrem are usually written in capital letters (REM and nonREM) but they will be in small case in this monograph to emphasize that they are not abbreviations but complete words referring to sleep states.

POLYGRAPHIC SLEEP

An all-night sleep pattern is recorded in the following manner. A standard EEG machine registers not only the scalp EEG but also eye movements between electrodes near each eye and the muscle activity between electrodes just medial to each mandibular body. For purposes of standardization, technical details of recording have been ritualized by a committee headed by Rechtschaffen and Kales (1968).

After the electrodes are applied, the light extinguished, and the door separating the sleeping room from the EEG technician closed, the normal subject drifts into sleep within a few minutes. The waking voluntary eye movements which make huge deflections in the electrooculogram disappear and the high level of muscle activity decreases. The background alpha rhythm disappears and the subject enters nonrem stage 1. With the appearance of sleep spindles and K-complexes, the subject enters nonrem stage 2. The K-complex, consisting of an initial negative wave followed by a positive wave, sometimes follows a sudden environmental stimulus such as a noise. Other K-complexes follow internal autonomic events such as bladder or gastrointestinal contractions (Johnson and Karpan, 1968). The sleep spindle is a burst of 12 to 15 cps activity lasting over one-half second. The term *spindle* relates to the spindle-shaped envelope of this sigma paroxysm. The sleep spindle, which shows remarkable phylogenetic stability, is generated by thalamocortical interrelations and disappears, at least temporarily, following lesions in the ipsilateral ventrolateral thalamus (Jurko and Andy, 1965). As nonrem sleep progresses, delta activity becomes more and more predominant and the sleeper enters nonrem stage 3 and then stage 4.

After about two hours of nonrem sleep, the sleeper rather abruptly enters rem sleep. The EEG changes to a relatively low voltage, mixed frequency pattern, and the chin EMG markedly decreases its activity up to a minute before the first conjugate eye movements occur. Frequently a burst of theta activity heralds the onset of a rem period (Dement, 1967). The theta waves which occur during rem sleep sometimes have a notch on the rising or falling phase to give the picture of sawteeth (Schwartz and Fischgold, 1960). These sawtooth waves, which are characteristic of rem sleep, frequently occur during or just before an eye movement (Berger et al., 1963). When the eyes move, the dipole moment of the electric charge on the retina and on the vascular epithelium behind the retina generates a potential which can be recorded by electrodes near the eye. These conjugate eye movements occur through all sizes of arcs in any direction and start from whatever position the eyes are in as a result of the preceding movement (Dement, 1964). Jacobs et al. (1971a) found that 25 to 35 percent of eye movements were in the vertical plane, 55 to 65 in the oblique plane, and 5 to 15 percent in the horizontal plane. While they report that the eye movements of rem sleep are unlike any eye movements recorded during wakefulness, others have described somewhat similar eye movements during periods of recalled visual imagery or "daydreaming" (Lorens and Darrow, 1962; Reyher and Morishige, 1969). Figure 1 presents polygraphic records from waking, rem sleep, and some nonrem sleep stages.

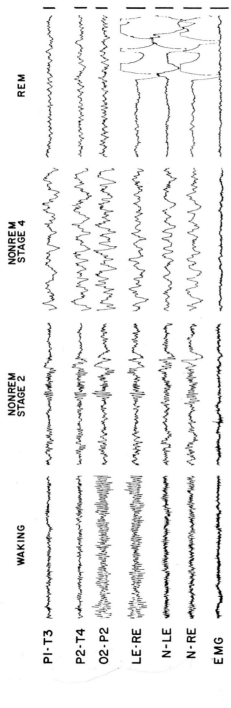

Figure 1. Samples from an all-night polygraphic recording. The top three channels monitor the EEG; the next three, eye movements; and the bottom channel is the electromyogram from the chin muscles. Some EEG rhythms come through on the eye channels during nonrem sleep and do not represent eye movement. The EEG during rem sleep contains intermittent theta activity. LE: lateral to the left eye, N: nasion.

Periods of nonrem and rem sleep alternate during the night. After the first long nonrem period, the cyclicity of this alternation averages about 90 minutes. The typical subject obtains most of his stage 4 during his first nonrem period. Nonrem periods in the early morning hours mainly consist of stage 2. Rem sleep also changes during the course of the night. The first rem period is shorter and has fewer eye movements than later rem periods (Goodenough et al., 1965: Verdone, 1965). Four to six rem periods occur during a night, making a fifth to a quarter of the total sleep time.

The polygraphic record produced by a complete night of sleep is rather long. At a paper speed of 15 mm/sec, the standard slow speed of sleep recording, eight hours of sleep produces a record which is over 400 meters long. This record is broken into 20-second epochs, and each epoch is scored as waking, rem sleep, or one of the nonrem sleep stages according to specific criteria. Table III lists some of the major criteria used in classifying these stages. The pamphlet edited by Rechtschaffen and Kales (1968) amplifies these criteria and gives examples, exceptions, and borderline cases. Most human sleep studies now follow the recommendations promulgated in this booklet which is available at no cost (except to the U.S. taxpayer) from the U.C.L.A. Brain Information Service.

TABLE III

SLEEP STAGE SCORING CRITERIA

Stage W: The EEG contains alpha activity associated with quiet wakefulness or low voltage activity with active wakefulness. The EMG has a high level of activity and there are frequent voluntary eye movements.

Stage 1: The EEG shows less than half the epoch occupied by alpha waves. No spindles or K-complexes occur in the EEG record. Occasional slow, rolling eye movements occur.

Stage 2: The EEG record shows K-complexes and bursts of 12 to 15 cycles per second rhythm and contains less than 20 percent delta activity. There are no eye movements.

Stage 3: The EEG contains between 20 and 50 percent of the epoch occupied by delta activity. There are no eye movements.

Stage 4: The EEG contains over 50 percent of the epoch occupied by delta activity. There may be spindle activity superimposed on the delta activity. There are no eye movements.

Stage REM: The EEG is relatively low voltage, mixed frequency activity with bursts of theta rhythm and saw-tooth waves. Conjugate rapid eye movements occur. The chin EMG reaches its lowest amplitude.

Many scoring difficulties arise from distinguishing the presence or absence of delta activity. When approximately 20 percent of an epoch is occupied by delta waves, some scorers might call that epoch stage 2 and some stage 3. Similarly, when approximately 50 percent of an epoch is taken up by delta activity, scorers have trouble differentiating stages 3 and 4 (Monroe, 1969). The latter problem is handled by some workers the same way Alexander untied the Gordian knot; they lump stages 3 and 4 together and call it high voltage slow sleep or delta sleep. Occasionally, difficulty arises separating W from nonrem stage 1, but spindles and K-complexes readily differentiate nonrem stages 1 and 2. Some workers report stage 2 latency, time from turning off the light to the first spindle or K-complex, rather than sleep latency, time to first stage 1, as a more reliable measure of the time it takes a subject to fall to a specific level of sleep. Attempts to score sleep stages by computer techniques have only been partially successful (Larsen and Walter, 1970; Lessard and Paschall, 1970; Roessler et al., 1970). Reports based solely upon computer scored all-night polygraphic records will not be considered in this book since the degree of correlation between human and machine scoring may vary with experimental manipulations (for example see Itil, 1969, 1970).

I would like to emphasize that the stages of nonrem sleep are obviously arbitrary subdivisions, while the rem and nonrem division of sleep is based on many physiologic differences. One could make the cutoff between stages 3 and 4 60 percent delta activity rather than 50 percent. This would produce more stage 3 and less stage 4, but little or no psychophysiologic information would be lost by this manuever. The identification of an epoch as rem or as nonrem sleep is based on three separate polygraphic measurements, and no single adjustment of scoring rules could significantly change the overall rem percentage. Despite the arbitrary nature of the nonrem subdivisions, the amount of stage 3 and stage 4 sleep gives a general, comparative value of the amount of delta activity occurring during a night or during a nonrem period.

NORMAL SLEEP PATTERNS

Several studies utilizing these techniques have described the normal sleep patterns of different groups. As summarized in Table IV, about 20 to 25 percent of a night's sleep is spent in the rem state. A very slight decrease in rem percentage and a somewhat larger decline in nonrem stage 4 may occur with increasing age. The most marked age effect is the decrease in total sleep time. This effect has been noted in nonpolygraphic studies of larger groups of subjects who estimate their own sleep time (Tune 1967, 1968). As a matter of fact, decreasing sleep time with age is an observation from time immemorium, summarized by Melville (1851):

> Old age is always wakeful; as if the longer linked with life the less man has to do with aught that looks like death. Among sea-commanders, the old greybeards will oftenest leave their berths to visit the night-cloaked deck. It was so with Ahab. . . . [This quotation is continued in the next chapter.]

An important technical detail in these studies of normal sleep patterns is the first night effect. The first night a subject sleeps in the laboratory he spends more time awake, has a decreased rem percentage, and has a longer latency to the first period of delta sleep and to the first rem period than on subsequent nights (Agnew et al., 1966; Mendels and Hawkins, 1967; Schmidt and Kaelbling, 1971). This slightly disturbed sleep pattern is thought to result from the anxiety associated with the unfamiliar experimental situation. All the studies of Table IV eliminated the first night of sleep in the laboratory from the final sleep stage percentages. Other environmental effects, such as daytime exercise (Baekeland, 1970), thirst (Koulack, 1970), or naps (Karacan et al., 1970b), can interfere with the polygraphic sleep pattern. Attempts to define normative sleep data are complicated by complex sleep adjustments to poorly understood environmental variables (Natani et al., 1970; Naitoh et al., 1970).

Table IV presents the average sleep patterns of different age groups; the extremes of normal sleep are quite wide. Jones and Oswald (1968) encountered two men who claimed they slept only two to three hours per night. These individuals appeared vigorous and restless. Their wives corroborated that their husbands slept less than three hours per night and only occasionally napped on weekends. Studied in the laboratory, the men slept an average of 2 hours and 45 minutes per night. Of the sleep they obtained, 1.9 percent was spent in nonrem stage 1, 24.5 percent in stage 2, 25.4 in stage 3, and 23.8 in stage 4. Rem percentage was 23.5. Hartmann and his co-

TABLE IV
SLEEP PATTERNS IN NORMAL MAN

	N	Average Age	Sleep Time	W	REM	Sleep Stage Percentages 1	2	3	4	Reference
Preadolescent males	18	9.5	565 min	1.5	24.3	6.1	44.2	5.9	17.9	Ross et al. (1968)
Young adult males	16	24.2	—	0.9	24.1	5.4	48.7	7.7	13.2	Williams et al. (1964)
Young adult females	16	23.9	451	1.1	21.9	5.9	48.0	6.9	16.2	Williams et al. (1966)
Adult males	12	33.9	—	2.4	21.9	7.5	53.0	5.5	9.6	Agnew and Webb (1968a)
Middle aged males	16	54.1	436	4.1	22.8	10.9	51.1	8.4	2.7	Agnew et al. (1967)
Elderly (both sexes)	16	63.4	—	9.9	20.4	11.9	50.6	4.5	2.7	Agnew and Webb (1968b)
Aged males	16	80.2	365.8	—	20.1	4.2	53.9	17.2	4.5	Kahn and Fisher (1969)
Aged females	16	76.7	383.0	—	18.0	2.6	63.4	10.4	5.6	Kahn et al. (1970)

workers (1971) collected through newspaper advertisements individuals who claimed to sleep less than 6 or more than 9 hours per night. The short sleepers were hardworking, conformist, mildly compulsive, and "establishment oriented." The long sleepers seemed anxious and depressed, and several openly admitted they used sleep as a defense from the pressures of life. In the sleep laboratory the long sleepers averaged 514 minutes of sleep while the age-matched short sleepers averaged only 330 minutes of sleep. The total stage 4 sleep in minutes was similar in the two groups, but, of course, the long sleepers had a decreased stage 4 percentage. Stage 3 percentage was also lower in the long sleepers. Rem percentage was similar in the two groups.

SLEEP OF INFANTS

The sleep of the normal human infant can be divided into two types. One type is characterized by no eye or body movements and regular respirations while the other type is associated with eye and body movements, irregular respiration, and spontaneous sucking (Parmelee et al., 1968; Prechtl, 1970, 1972). The first type of sleep develops into nonrem sleep, the latter into rem. Sleep spindles first appear in the nonrem EEG record of the term infant at about one month of age (Lenard, 1970; Metcalf, 1970). Unlike the adult, the infant usually passes from wakefulness directly into rem sleep. At about three months of age the infant begins to show the adult pattern of falling from wakefulness into nonrem sleep (Metcalf, 1971). Eye movements during neonatal rem sleep are not identical to either eye movements of the waking newborn or of the adult rem state (Prechtl and Lenard, 1967). In the newborn, deep tendon monosyaptic reflexes become most active during nonrem sleep and are actually depressed during rem sleep (Prechtl et al., 1967). While one cannot test tendon reflexes during adult sleep without causing arousal, the monosynaptic H-reflex is absent during rem sleep (Hodes and Dement, 1964). Tactile reflexes such as the palmar and plantar grasp reflexes and the palmomental reflex are well developed during rem but absent during nonrem sleep of the normal newborn (Lenard et al., 1968). The suck reflex is also prominent in rem sleep (Petre-Quadens, 1966). The Babinski response is approximately equal in wakefulness, rem, and nonrem in the normal neonate (Lenard et al., 1968). It has been suggested that the changes in both rem and nonrem EEG can determine conceptional age and neurological maturation in premature infants (Parmelee et al., 1968; Dreyfus-Brisac, 1970). The rem percentage of the term newborn is approximately 40 to 50 percent of the sleeping time (Roffwarg et al., 1966; Petre-Quadens, 1967), but technical difficulties prevent full agreement upon the rem percentage of the premature infant.

GROWTH HORMONE

Except for increases following hypoglycemia, exercise, and psychic stress, human growth hormone maintains a relatively low, constant serum level during wakefulness (reviewed by Catt, 1970). A peak of growth hormone activity occurs shortly after sleep onset and coincides with the first nightly appearance of slow wave sleep, nonrem stages three and four (Takahashi et al., 1968; Parker et al., 1969). Unlike during waking, growth hormone release from the anterior pituitary concomitant with slow wave sleep is not increased by previous exercise (Zir et al., 1971) nor is it blocked by glucose infusion (Parker and Rossman, 1971). Deprivation studies suggest that growth hormone secretion is related both to sleep onset itself and to the delta activity of nonrem stages 3 and 4 (Sassin et al., 1969; Karacan et al., 1971). The possible occurrence of stress-induced growth hormone release complicates phylogenetic and ontogenetic comparisons of the findings that no clear relation exists between sleep patterns and serum growth hormone levels in restrained monkeys (Sassin et al., 1971) and newborn infants from whom blood was collected for assay by puncture of the heel (Shaywitz et al., 1971). While other hormones have not been studied as thoroughly as growth hormone, some preliminary studies link rem periods with increased secretion of cortisol (Hellman et al., 1970), testosterone (Evans et al., 1971), anti-diuretic hormone (Mandell et al., 1966), and luteinizing hormone (Rubin et al., 1972).

Chapter 2

MENTAL ACTIVITY DURING SLEEP

And thus upon a night, there came a vision to Sir Launcelot, and charged him, in remission of his sins, to haste him unto Almesbury: And by then thou come there, thou shalt find Queen Guenever dead. And therefore take thy fellows with thee, and purvey them of an horse bier, and fetch thou the corpse of her, and bury her by her husband, the noble King Arthur. So this avision came to Sir Launcelot thrice in one night.

MALORY, *Le Morte D'Arthur*

DREAMS

THE twentieth century began with Sigmund Freud's *Interpretation of Dreams*. In his neurologic practice, Freud had urged his hysteric and neurotic patients to delve into their own thoughts to uncover hidden emotional problems. In the subsequent free associations these patients frequently brought up material from their dreams. Stimulated by the importance of these dreams in the patients' emotional lives, Freud began analyzing his own dreams as well as those told to him by his friends and some dreams of history and literature. Freud thought that more important than the manifest content of the dream story was the underlying or latent content. He suggested that the unconscious mind produced thematic elements which were too traumatic and emotional for the conscious mind to deal with so that a hypothetical censor converted these themes into symbols. Each dream contained events of the preceding day, the day residue, and events or themes from the sleeper's past life, particularly his childhood. The symbolic drama of the dream provided wish fulfillment and catharsis, particularly for the unconscious. Freud pointed out that several different themes can be pursued in the same dream with each character in the dream representing two or more characters of waking life. *The Interpretation of Dreams* is Freud's great work and will always remain one of the great books of modern man.

Of course many of Freud's ideas existed in the science and literature which preceded him, but his was the first major synthesis of these ancient ideas. In his *Parliament of Birds,* Geoffrey Chaucer clearly described wish fulfillment and hinted at the concept of day residue:

> When the weary hunter sleeps, anon his mind returns to the wood; the judge dreams how his cases be sped, and the carter how his carts go; the rich dream of gold, the knight fights his foes; the sick man dreams he drinks of the tun, the lover that he has his lady.

C.G. Jung developed further Freud's idea of the unconscious. Each individual's unconscious has some elements in common with the unconscious of each other individual, said Jung. This collective unconscious has developed through brain evolution just as bodily characteristics of the human species have developed through evolution of the rest of the body. Dreams serve as an approach to the collective unconscious as well as to those portions of each individual's unconscious which are related to his own personal environmental experiences. Jung compared dreams and myths from cultures which had little or no contact with one another and found certain symbols in common. Erich Fromm (1951) suggested that Freud's approach to dream interpretation emphasized that all dreams are of an irrational nature while Jung emphasized that dreams are revelations of higher wisdom. Fromm expressed the view that "dreams partake of both our irrational and our rational nature, and it is the aim of the art of dream interpretation to understand when our better self and when our animal nature makes itself heard in the dream" (p. 147). Calvin Hall (1953) believed that the interpretations of Freud and his followers had been colored by their analysis of the dreams of neurotic patients. Collecting dream reports from hundreds of normal persons, he found that most dreams had an unpleasant quality to them and that they usually involved one of these basic conflicts:

> (1) the "eternal triangle"; the dreamer competing for the love of someone of the opposite sex against someone of the same sex; sometimes the dream explicitly identifies these two people as the dreamer's parents;
> (2) independence versus security, with dreams alternating between the dreamer going out on his own or falling back into a dependency upon family or society;

(3) conflict of sex roles;

(4) fear of death; and

(5) moral conflict, with the dreamer suffering punishment for transgressions of the previous day or for deeds or thoughts contrary to society's moral code which occur in the dream itself.

These and other workers vociferously criticized Freud's concepts of the censor and his idea that each dream must represent wish fulfillment. The unconscious mind may use symbols at all times, and one need not hypothesize a mythical entity which converts unconscious thinking into hidden meanings which can be understood by one part of the mind but not another. If dreams are meant as merely fulfillment of wishes, one wonders why such a high percentage of them are so unpleasant. Freud was obviously hard pressed to explain this paradox when he offered these two rather flimsy suggestions. Unpleasant dreams might represent masochistic desires to suffer or could represent the dreamer's wish that Freud's theory is not true. A person wishes Freud's idea of wish fulfillment in dreams to be incorrect; therefore he dreams an unpleasant dream.

At this point we must mention the prophetic dream. One cannot talk about sleep and dreaming for long without someone bringing up a prophetic dream from his own experience. For example, my secretary who typed this chapter brought it to me with the story that her mother has dreams which predict the future. Prophetic dreams are frequent in ancient history; the Bible relates several. Senator Arthur V. Watkins in his memoirs (1969) relates this modern prophetic dream:

> Only a few nights before I had had a dream in which I had been named to serve on the Select Committee to consider the charges against Senator Joseph R. McCarthy of Wisconsin. In my dream, still worse, I had been made Chairman of the Committee. So realistic was the nightmare that I had awakened, struggling to free myself from its unpleasant implications.

One might classify prophetic dreams into three categories: after the fact, statistical, and inner knowledge. An after-the-fact dream is easiest to explain. Many years after an event, a participant from his rich dream life builds the memory of a dream which, taken at its face value, clearly predicted the event. For example, after William the Conqueror had successfully invaded England in 1066, his mother recalled that when pregnant with the future Norman conqueror she had dreamed that a great tree grew out of her body and spread its branches across the sea (Slocombe, 1959). Many ancient historical dreams are after the fact. A statistical dream is one which is dreamed quite often but is only remembered after the prediction comes true. From the work of Hall and others, we know that dreamers frequently portray the death of loved ones in their dreams. This is remembered vividly only when the actual death occurs closely following the prophetic dream. Senator Watkins' dream may be of this nature. The Senate was swirling with rumors and hints of the organization of a committee to investigate Senator McCarthy, and it is not unlikely that many senators had dreams similar to Watkins'; only his was remembered because only his was prophetic.

The problem of inner-knowledge prophetic dreams is more complex. Despite the fantasy nature of much dream material, sometimes one is closer to reality in dreams than during wakefulness. The Bible relates two dreams of Joseph which predicted this small boy would surpass his father and his brothers:

Now Israel love Joseph more than all his children, because he was the son of his old age; and he made him a coat of many colors. And when his brethren saw that their father loved him more than all his brethren, they hated him and could not speak peaceably unto him. And Joseph dreamed a dream, and he told it his brethren and they hated him yet the more. And he said unto them, Hear, I pray you, this dream which I have dreamed: For, behold, we were binding sheaves in the field, and lo, my sheaf arose, and also stood upright; and, behold, your sheaves stood round about, and made obeisance to my sheaf. And his brethren said to him, Shalt thou indeed reign over us? Or shalt thou indeed have dominion over us? And they hated him yet the more for his dreams, and for his words. And he dreamed yet another dream, and told it his brethren, and said, Behold, I have dreamed a dream more; and behold, the sun and the moon and the eleven stars made obeisance to me. And he told it to his father, and to his brethren: and his father rebuked him, and said unto him, What is this dream that thou hast dreamed? Shall I and thy mother and thy brethren indeed come to bow down ourselves to thee to the earth?

GENESIS 37:3-10

Note how the symbolism of the dream is instantly interpreted by these ordinary shepherds without need of psychiatrist or shaman. These were prophetic dreams which "came true"; Joseph rose to prominence in Egypt and his brothers bowed down before him. The prophetic character of these dreams might be explained by assuming that during waking life the stronger brothers awed young Joseph; yet during sleep he realized he was more ambitious and intelligent than they and had a good chance of accomplishing much more than they ever would.

The ability to see oneself more clearly during sleep than during waking was utilized in ancient Greece by the cult of Aesculapius. The Aesculapian priest-physicians directed each patient to sleep in the Temple of Aesculapius and to dream about his illness. The dream was then interpreted to indicate diagnosis and treatment. This type of medical treatment was apparently common in the ancient world. In his review of the religions of ancient and primitive peoples, Hays (1967) reported dream healing or dream divination in the ancient civilizations of the Egyptians, the Babylonians, the Maltese, and the Celtics as well as among many modern African and Amerindian tribes. Gauguin's painting reproduced in Figure 2 may represent Tahitian natives sleeping in the presence of one of their idols so that this god can influence their dreams. The modern counterpart of the Aesculapians and similar cults which utilize the dream to reach inner knowledge is the frequently told story, probably apocryphal, of the psychoanalyst who correctly diagnosed an intracranial arteriovenous malformation when his patient dreamed about waterfalls. During waking the slight sound of the malformation went unnoticed, but in sleep it induced dreams of waterfalls. This method is not universally successful; a patient of mine who had mental changes associated with adrenal insufficiency told me that Jesus appeared to him in a dream and told him his illness was due to appendicitis, and he should have an appendectomy (Freemon and Drake, 1967, case 8). He didn't even have abdominal pain.

If prophetic dreams existed which truly predicted future events on a basis other than the pattern of past events, we should be forced to change all our ideas about causation. The clear and unequivocal occurrence of truly prophetic dreams would rock science to its foundations.

SLEEP MENTATION

When a person first learns that there are two types of sleep, he

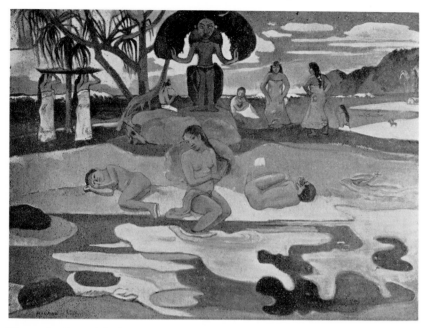

Figure 2. Gauguin's *Day of the God (Mahana no Atus)*. Many ancient and modern primitive cultures practiced the art of religious dream incubation. Reproduced with the courtesy of the Art Institute of Chicago.

usually asks one of two questions. Either he asks which type is "deepest," a surprisingly complex question which is considered later, or he inquires which type of sleep is "dreaming" sleep. The dreams discussed in the previous section are extracted from the sleeper either by his memory the next day of his previous night's mental activity or his written condensation of his sleep mentation after spontaneous awakening. A new dimension to the mental activity of the sleeper has been obtained by an experimenter awakening a person from a specific sleep stage identified by polygraphic criteria and asking him what was going through his mind immediately prior to the arousal. Of course, sometimes the sleeper replies that nothing was in his mind; his mind was blank. Occasionally he states that something was in his mind, but he can give no details of it; it has slipped from memory during the process of awakening. Sometimes the person denies he was asleep and claims he was lying awake, thinking. Usually, however, the sleeper gives some mental content that he claims was present in his mind at the moment of awakening. The type of mentation reported following awakenings from nonrem sleep usually differs qualitatively from rem sleep reports.

Awakenings from nonrem sleep produce reports of ongoing mental activity characterized by specific thoughts and devoid of dramatic story content with minimal sensory imagery. Here is an example non-rem mentation report obtained by Foulkes (1962):

> I was thinking about this phone call I got from home tonight. I got a long-distance call from home, and my parents were very angry with me because I haven't written. They really gave me heck for about 20 minutes on the phone tonight, which bothered me no end. I had been thinking that this last time you rang the bell, and I had a very unpleasant feeling about it. I was rehearsing their conversation in my mind.

Some degree of mental activity occurs in about half of stage 4 and two thirds of stage 3 awakenings. Arousals from nonrem stage 2 produce reports of thinking about 70 percent of the time (Pivik and Foulkes, 1968). The mental activity occurring at sleep onset, during nonrem stage 1, shows some similarities to rem mentation (Foulkes and Vogel, 1965; Vogel et al., 1966). A small minority of people suffer severe nightmares during nonrem stages 3 and 4; they may awaken screaming and confused but be unable to relate the mental activity that so terrified them (Broughton, 1968; Fisher et al., 1970). Most people who claim they have suffered a nightmare, however, have suffered anxiety during a rem period.

Subjects awakened from rem sleep report ongoing visual images forming a coherent drama. The length of the story approximates the length of the rem period (Dement and Wolpert, 1958). The visual experiences are usually in color (Kahn et al., 1962) and are accompanied to a lesser extent by auditory stimuli and other senses. One of the most characteristic aspects of rem mentation is that despite the marked fantasy nature of the story material, the sleeper accepts this unreal behavior as perfectly natural. For example, the sleeper fails to recognize the incompatibility of his own embarrassment with others' casual acceptance of his being at work or school stark naked. Rem mentation parallels nonrem mentation in that it either rapidly fades from memory completely or is markedly distorted unless it is rehearsed in the mind after awakening (Baekeland and Lasky, 1968).

Up to this point we have described rem and nonrem mentation

without recourse to the word dream. Like so many other words, dream has taken on a completely different meaning for different subgroups of people and has almost completely lost any value for communication between members of different scientific subdisciplines. If one defines dream as a story-like visual experience with the dreamer failing to recognize its fantasy components as unreal, then dreaming is restricted to rem periods. But if one defines a dream simply as mental activity during sleep, then dreaming occurs during nonrem as well as rem periods. Table V summarizes some of the many studies of recall after awakening from rem and nonrem sleep states and shows how the percentage of dream reports obtained depends upon the definition of dreaming. A meeting of psychologists attempted to formulate a definition of dreaming, but only reached the unhelpful consensus that each investigator should use his own definition (Clemente, 1967). The difficulty of this area was exemplified by the title of one of the papers presented: "When is a dream is a dream is a dream?" (Berger, 1967). Some of the confusion of trying to mix the physiologic concept of rem sleep with the psychological concept of dreaming can be seen from these quotations:

> Dreaming occurs most frequently during REM states, but it can also occur during NREM states of sleeping and even waking. REM states, therefore, seem to be only predisposing conditions for dreaming. (Lehmann, 1969)

> Of course, the patient may have had dream periods during nonREM stages of sleep; however these are not measureable and could not be included in the total dream time. (Freedman et al., 1969)

In the remainder of this monograph we will try to stick to these definitions: (1) Rem mentation is the mental activity which occurs during rem sleep and is sampled by waking the sleeper during the rem state and asking him what was going through his mind; (2) nonrem mentation is the mental activity occurring during nonrem sleep, sampled by waking the sleeper during nonrem sleep; (3) a dream is the narrative someone reports the following day of some mental activity occurring under the conditions of sleep, e.g. "I had an interesting dream last night." One finds, of course, that most dreams reported in this way are probably reports of rem mentation. For example, most of the dreams recorded by Freud in his *Interpretation of Dreams* are probably products of the mentation occurring during rem sleep; several, however, could have occurred during Freud's nonrem sleep state, an example being Freud's dream of a single word, *autodidasker*.

With this background we can again consider the question, during which of the sleep states does dreaming occur? This turns out to be a falsely simple question. Many people with a peripheral interest in sleep research cannot grasp the difference between dreaming and sleep mentation. When addressing such a group, say a lay audience, I find it necessary to equate the rem state with "dreaming sleep." I always feel foolish when I do, though, because this is a gross oversimplification. The concepts of dreaming developed by Freud, Jung, Fromm, Hall, and others exist independently of polygraphic research. Fromm (1951), for example, defined a dream as "any kind of mental activity under the condition of sleep" (p. 47), a definition which includes nonrem mental experiences. On the other hand, research into psychologic differences between rem and nonrem mentation can complement physiologic descriptions of sleep and perhaps increase our knowledge of the physiologic events which underlie psychologic processes. There is more than one way to examine the mind at night.

If you awaken in the morning with dream-like thoughts in your mind, you may wish to know if this sleep mentation comes from the rem or the nonrem state. You may be able to identify the type of mentation by its content. If your thoughts consisted of the rehashing of an idea with little sensory imagery, then they probably originated during nonrem sleep. If your thoughts formed a fantastic drama, then you probably awakened from a rem period. Many or most of the sleep thoughts occurring upon awakening will not be classifiable into rem and nonrem categories on this basis. The male reader has the additional information provided by penile tumescence. If you awaken with an erection, you are probably awakening from a rem period. Only polygraphic recording, of course, can unequivocally identify the sleep states.

An interesting example of sleep mentation is given by Eric Ambler in his *Epitaph for a Spy* (1938). The narrator, a hapless language teacher named Joseph Vadassy has been trapped into spying on his fellow hotel guests by the counter-intelligence agent Beghin:

> The night was getting cold. I went back to bed. Then, as my eyes closed once more, a new fear began to gather in my mind, turning over and

TABLE V
SLEEP MENTATION AND DREAMING

Awakenings from:					
Rem		Nonrem			
Total Number	Dream Recall	Total Number	Dream Recall	Definition of Dreaming	Authors
27	74%	23	7%	"detailed dream description"	Aserinsky and Kleitman (1955)
51	88%	19	0%	self-definition by each subject	Dement (1955)
191	79%	161	7%	"coherent, fairly detailed description"	Dement and Kleitman (1957)
91	69%	99	34%	"a dream recalled in some detail"	Goodenough et al. (1959)
20	60%	30	3%	self-definition by each subject	Jouvet et al. (1960)
67	85%	21	24%	self-definition by each subject	Wolpert (1960)
108	87%	136	74%	"any item of specific content"	Foulkes (1962)
108	82%	136	54%	"visual, auditory, or kinesthetic imagery"	Foulkes (1962)
186	86%	96	23%	"specific content of mental experience"	Rechtschaffen et al. (196)
108	81%	134	7%	"any sensory imagery with . . . progression of the mental activity"	Kales et al. (1967)
46	74%	150	58%	"a DF rating of at least 2"	Larson and Foulkes (1969)
84	95%	84	81%	"fragmentary reports with little content"	Castaldo and Shevrin (1970)

over, growing bigger, a terrible possibility. Supposing one of the guests left the hotel? It might easily happen. Tomorrow, Herr Vogel or Monsieur Duclos or Roux and his blonde, any of them, might say: "I have decided to leave at once." For all I knew one of them might already have his luggage packed to leave in the morning. What could I do to stop him, Supposing I were wrong about Koche and Schimler. Supposing that the Americans or the Swiss or the English were spies. They would slip through my fingers. No use to tell myself that I would deal with the question when it arose. That might be too late. What exactly should I do? Quickly now! Imagine they're all going, leaving you here alone in the morning. What would you do? Get a pistol from Beghin. Yes, that was it, get a pistol from Beghin. Stand no nonsense. "Stand where you are or I'll fill your guts with lead." Ten rounds in the magazine. "One for each of you." No, eight rounds in the magazine. It depends on the type of pistol. I should need two.

I threw back the clothes and sat up. At this rate I should be a lunatic by morning. I went to the washbasin and sluiced my face with water. I must, I told myself, have been dreaming. But I knew perfectly well that I had not been to sleep.

The Hotel Reserve on the French Riviera was not equipped wtih polygraph machines in 1938, but I would wager that Joseph Vadassy was asleep when those thoughts ran through his mind; in fact, I would wager he was in nonrem sleep. The repetitive nature of the thoughts, the lack of visual imagery, the loosening of reality without the construction of a fantastic drama, all point toward typical nonrem mentation occurring just after sleep onset.

INCORPORATION OF ENVIRONMENTAL STIMULI

Environmental stimuli can be incorporated into ongoing sleep mentation. Freud himself related a dream of riding a horse that he thought was induced by a painful scrotal boil. In later editions of his *Dreams* Freud described a night when loud church bells awakened his wife but caused Freud to dream about the death of the Pope. History and literature abound with dreams influenced by such environmental stimuli as the clump, clump, clump of Captain Ahab's ivory peg leg:

Habitually the silent steersman would watch the cabin scuttle; and ere long the old man would emerge, griping at the iron banister to help his crippled way. Some considering touch of humanity was in him; for at times like these he usually abstained from patrolling the quarterdeck; because to his wearied mates, seeking repose within six inches of his ivory heel, such would have been the reverberating crack and din of that bony step that their dreams would have been of the crunching teeth of sharks. (Melville, 1851)

Studies of polygraphically monitored sleep have provided anecdotes suggesting that auditory, visual, and somesthetic stimuli can be incorporated into ongoing rem mentation. Dement and Wolpert (1958) found that dripping water on exposed skin, flashing a light, or sounding a tone during a rem period resulted in incorporation of these stimuli into rem mentation 42, 23, and 9 percent of the time respectively. An example of fairly direct incorporation is quoted:

> The S was sleeping on his stomach. His back was uncovered. An eye movement period started and after it had persisted for 10 minutes, cold water was sprayed on his back. Exactly 30 seconds later he was awakened. The first part of the dream involved a rather complex description of acting in a play. Then, "I was walking behind the leading lady when she suddenly collapsed and water was dripping on her face. I ran over to her and felt water dripping on my back and head. The roof was leaking. I was very puzzled why she fell down and decided some plaster must have fallen on her. I looked up and there was a hole in the roof. I dragged her over to the side of the stage and began pulling the curtains. Just then I woke up." (Dement and Wolpert, 1958)

Berger (1963) played familiar and unfamiliar names during rem periods and found occasions when the names were directly heard in the ongoing rem mentation, when the person with the familiar name appeared as a character in the drama, and when an object appeared in the drama which rhymed with the auditory stimulus. An example of the latter is an appearance of a rabbit in the narrative after the repetition of the word Robert. Koulack (1969) stimulated the sleeper's wrist electrically during rem periods and found a significant incorporation of this stimulus into ongoing rem mentation. He obtained the highest incorporation percentage, 64, when the stimulus was applied three minutes after the beginning of the rem period, and the sleeper was awakened three minutes later. The incorporation could be direct: "I felt a pinch in my hand. Electrical impulse. With this electrical impulse I got up out of bed and I sat near a desk. I looked at the time and it was 5 o'clock and I went back to bed again. And the phone rang and I realized it was just a dream." The phone ringing was the representation in the ongoing rem mentation of the awakening buzzer. Other descriptions of rem mentation were judged by the author to be examples of indirect incorporation: "I dreamt that I had a snake on my bed in the lab, and it was a long black snake, and I had to call you up because I didn't know what to do." Several other studies have examined more subtle effects of external stimuli on ongoing sleep mentation. For example, Castaldo and Holzman (1967, 1969) found that a recording of the sleeper's own voice played during the rem state produced rem mentation in which the central character of the drama was active and assertive while a recording of another person's voice saying the same words produced rem mentation in which the central character was in a passive position. In summary, there is little doubt that ongoing rem mentation can be affected by environmental stimuli. Nonrem sleep has not been studied in this regard extensively though a few anecdotes exist suggesting that auditory and other stimuli can be directly incorporated into ongoing nonrem mentation (Foulkes, 1967).

PSYCHOPHYSIOLOGIC PARALLELISM

The relation of rem mentation to movements of the sleeper, particularly eye movements, remains unclear. Dement and Wolpert (1958) and Berger and Oswald (1962b) reported that those rem periods with the most eye movements had the most visual imagery. Since the later rem periods of the night have more eye movements and more vivid mentation than earlier ones, many interpretations of this relationship between eye movements and mentation are possible besides the suggestion that more eye movements result from the sleeper looking at more vivid action. Quite a bit of anecdotal evidence suggests, however, that the eye movements of rem sleep do result from the sleeper moving his eyes in response to the changes of visual imagery in his ongoing sleep mentation. In his summary of this problem of psychophysiologic parallelism, Wolpert (1968) points out that only a minority of experimental subjects have the necessary combination of introspective and expressive abilities to register their internal subjective experience and to describe it adequately to the experimenter. Dement and Kleitman (1957) awakened sleepers after specific eye movements of rem sleep and sometimes found close parallel mental activity. A subject observed to have a series of horizontal eye movements, for example, related that his rem mentation had included two people throwing tomatoes at each other. Roffwarg et al. (1962) provided further examples such as the individual whose rem period concluded with five upward eye movements and who related his dream of slowly climbing steps, glancing up at each step. Utilizing strict separation of the person who interrogated the sleeper from the person who monitored the polygraphic data, Roffwarg and his co-workers found in a significant number of awakenings, a correlation between direction and type of eye movement with the visual imagery occurring just before arousal. Moskowitz and Berger (1969) and Jacobs et al. (1971a) were unable to confirm these results, but they give no information about how extensive was the interrogation nor how introspective and cooperative were the subjects. An example given by Dement (1964) points out how the interrogator and the subject must probe the rem mentation to obtain enough information to predict eye movement:

> Subject (giving his dream): "I was lying on my back on a bed in the laboratory. There were two people outside in the hall and I was listening to them, trying to hear what they were saying. Just as I woke up, one of them started to open the door and I looked to see who it was."
> Experimenter: "How long were you listening?"
> S: "Oh, a minute or two."
> E: "What were you looking at while you were listening?"
> S: "Well, I was lying on my back with my head turned toward the wall and I was just staring toward the wall."
> E: "What were the positions of the bed and the door?"
> S: "The bed was against the wall on my right and the door was in the same wall a foot or so beyond the foot of the bed."

On the basis of these additional questions the interrogator predicted that the polygraphic record would show a long period of ocular quiescence and then an eye movement down and to the left, which was in fact the case. A high degree of correlation between mental activity during rem sleep and eye movements cannot be expected without close questioning of introspective subjects. Despite these frequent examples of eye movement and rem mentation correspondence, many workers feel that eye movements must be independent of mentation. Blind people whose rem mentation lack visual imagery were thought to have no eye movements during the regular cyclic recurrences of the rem state as judged by EEG and EMG criteria (Offenkrantz and

Wolpert, 1963; Berger, Olley, and Oswald, 1962), but later studies utilizing direct observation and mechanical rather than electrical measurement of eye movements have shown that the blind do have eye movements during rem sleep. The earlier results were due to loss of the corneoretinal potential in some individuals with retinal degeneration (Amadeo and Gomez, 1965; Gross et al., 1965). Most animal workers, observing frequent eye movements in normal and lesioned animals during rem sleep, have been unable to accept the "looking at a picture" hypothesis. Eye movements during rem sleep in experimental animals are discussed in the next chapter. Though nonrem mentation occasionally contains visual imagery, eye movements do not occur. The relationship between ongoing mentation and eye movements remains locked to anecdotal evidence.

Similar evidence relates body movements to rem mentation. Dement (1967) provides the best anecdote:

> One night I became aware that my wife's legs were twitching with unusual vigor. Being a sleep researcher to the core, I turned on the bed lamp and looked at her eyes which, naturally, were moving rapidly. Unable to resist, I aroused her and she recalled a dream of dancing a wild Viennese waltz.

Hobson and his co-workers (1965) have provided examples of apneic periods during rem sleep associated with fantasied respiratory difficulties in the simultaneous rem mentation.

OTHER ASPECTS OF REM MENTATION

Many other aspects of sleep mentation are under investigation. A number of investigators have examined the influence of evening activity on subsequent rem mentation (Baekeland et al., 1968; Witkin and Lewis, 1967; Cartwright et al., 1969; Hauri, 1970). Much rem mentation contains elements relating to the sleep laboratory, especially on the subject's first night (Dement et al., 1965; Domhoff and Kamiya, 1964b), and rem mentation as sampled in the sleep laboratory contains fewer sexual and aggressive narratives than the same subjects' dreams which they recall when sleeping at home (Domhoff and Kamiya, 1964a; Weisz and Foulkes, 1970). Orr et al. (1968) found that subjects trying to awaken themselves at specific times frequently had rem narratives concerning deadlines or traveling. Perhaps stimulated by Descartes' account of his three interrelated dreams of one night which determined his lifelong project to bring all human knowledge together without theoretical bias, a number of workers have awakened sleepers from several rem periods on the same night to investigate the relationship of the mentation of one rem period with that of the next (Rechtschaffen et al., 1963; Kramer et al., 1964). In general, later rem periods have much more vivid imagery and a more dramatic narrative than earlier rem periods (Domhoff and Kamiya, 1964c; Verdone, 1965; Goodenough et al., 1965). Ullman and Kripner (1970) have attempted to demonstrate that extrasensory perception can influence rem mentation. The mental activity which occurs during the rem sleep of children has been studied by Foulkes and co-workers (1969).

Both rem and nonrem mentation rapidly slip from memory unless rehearsed immediately upon awakening. It is not at all unusual in sleep research to have a subject deny any dreams or any interruption of his previous night's sleep to find to his surprise that he not only had vivid rem mentation but was awakened and reported his mentation to the investigator (see, for example, Baekeland and Lasky, 1968). Portnoff et al. (1966) awakened individuals several times per night and had them repeat a word. If the subjects stayed awake for five minutes before returning to sleep they could remember some of the words the next morning, but if they returned immediately to sleep they had no recollection for the words. The reader who wishes to increase his conscious awareness of what goes on in his own mind at night is advised to lie in bed a moment or two after awakening and try to remember what was running through his mind just before he woke. If he cannot remember the entire narrative sequence he can begin at the most recent event and work backwards until his memory gives out. Even when he feels quite confident of remembering the narrative, he should go over the events two or three more times. He should then record his mental experience on paper to avoid the problem which afflicted Otto Loewi. After mulling thoughts about nerve function all day, he fell asleep only to awaken with a clear idea of the experiment which could prove chemical transmission in the peripheral nervous system. He jotted down a note or two and then happily returned to sleep. He was terrified the next day, however, when he could not remember the experiment his sleeping mind had devised, nor could he decipher his notes. Luckily, the same dream occurred the next night, and he recorded it in detail.

Chapter 3

SLEEP OF ANIMALS

But ask now the beast, and they shall teach thee; and the fowls of the air, and they shall tell thee.

JOB 12:7

SLEEP PHYLOGENY

MOST mammals have two types of sleep. As in man, animal nonrem sleep has spindles and slow waves in the EEG and no eye movements. A low voltage, mixed frequency EEG and an abolition of tone in the posterior neck muscles occur during rem sleep. Except in those animals, such as armadillo and mole, who have poorly developed waking eye movements, conjugate eye movements accompany rem sleep. In some species postural changes characterize the two sleep states; for example, the cat has a sphinx-like posture during nonrem sleep, but the head drops to the forepaws as the animal enters rem sleep. Table VI summarizes several studies of the sleep of normal animals of different species. Each study involved 24-hour observation and/or polygraphic recording; all animals were unrestrained except the rhesus monkeys who were habituated to a restraint chair. None of the data of Table VI can be considered completely normative because no animal has yet been studied in its native habitat. Rem sleep has also been described in a large number of farm animals including lamb, pig, donkey, horse, goat, and cow by Ruckebush and his co-workers (1962, 1963, 1968). A long habituation period is needed before rem sleep can be observed in adult ungulates. Allison and Goff (1968) reported that the primitive spiny anteater, an egg laying mammal, had no rem sleep.

Some bird species also show rem sleep. The hawk and the falcon have brief periods of rem sleep which make up about 7 to 10 percent of the four to five hours of sleep that these birds obtain each night (Rojas-Ramirez and Tauber, 1970). Chickens and pigeons have even

TABLE VI

SLEEP OF MAMMALS

Species	Total Sleep per 24 Hours	Rem Percentage	Cycle Length	Reference
Man	8 hours	23%	90 min.	See Chapter 1
Chimpanzee	14	15	—	Bert et al. (1970)
	12	23	85	Freemon et al. (1971)
Rhesus	—	20	54	Weitzman et al. (1965)
	6	15	51	Kripke et al. (1968)
Cat	16	23	27	Delorme et al. (1964)
	14	28	26	Sterman et al. (1965)
	13	24	24	Ursin (1968)
Rat	13	20	9	Van Twyver (1969)
	—	16	14	Weiss and Roldan (1964)
Mouse	13	10	12	Van Twyver (1969)
	—	18	8	Weiss and Roldan (1964)
Hamster	14	23	12	Van Twyver (1969)
Squirrel	14	25	13	Van Twyver (1969)
Chinchilla	12	12	6	Van Twyver (1969)
Mole	8	25	10	Allison and Van Twyver (1970)
Opossum	19	29	23	Van Twyver and Allison (1970)
Rabbit	—	15	25	Weiss and Roldan (1964)
	7	11	42	Narebski et al. (1969)
Tree shrew	16	16	12	Berger et al. (1970)

a smaller amount of rem sleep (Klein et al., 1964; Hishikawa et al., 1969). The rem state must have either been present in the primitive reptile which gave rise to birds and mammals, or it must have evolved independently in these two orders. The study of sleep in reptiles and amphibians is complicated by the primitive forebrain of these species which lacks a structure homologous to the neocortex which gives rise to the scalp or cortical EEG of mammals. Nevertheless, some investigators have tentatively identified rem sleep in the lizard (Tauber et al., 1968) and the turtle (Vasilescu, 1970).

Some species, like man or the chimpanzee, are diurnal, active in the daytime and sleeping at night. Other species, galago is an example, are nocturnal, sleeping during the day and being active only at night. Other species show more complicated rest-activity cycles; the wild rabbit shows greatest activity about dawn and dusk with periods of relative inactivity between. A few animals show a rest activity cycle without any simple relationship to a circadian rhythm. The cat may sleep at any time, night or day, a habit which has given us the term cat nap. The rat, though generally more active at night, obtains his sleep in brief naps (Webb and Friedmann, 1971). The cat is the traditional species of neurophysiologic research. Most of the results discussed in the rest of this chapter were obtained from this species. However, the understanding of the circadian aspects of human sleep is unlikely to be aided by the study of cat sleep since the cat shows such a poorly developed circadian sleep rhythm.

ELECTRICAL ACTIVITY

During nonrem sleep in the cat and other species, slow waves and sleep spindles occur in cortex and in most subcortical locations. However, in the cat, low voltage fast activity occupies specific thalamic nuclei, pulvinar, pontine, and bulbar reticular formation (Jouvet 1962, 1967; Desiraju et al., 1966). Sleep spindles consist of bursts of 11 to 16 cps activity in cortex, thalamus, and midbrain reticular formation. Neurosurgical separation of thalamus and cortex from midbrain abolishes spindle activity caudal but not rostral to the lesion (Villablanca and Schlag, 1968). Thalamic spindles continue after decortication (Andersson et al., 1971b). Purpura (1969, 1972) relates the frequency of the spindle waves to the duration of the inhibitory postsynaptic potential in thalamic neurons. The cortical activity during nonrem sleep in subhuman primates is so similiar to the scalp activity of man that nonrem sleep in a number of primate species can be divided into four substages according to the Rechschaffen and Kales (1968) rules devised for man. These species include chimpanzee (Bert et al., 1970; Freemon et al., 1971), rhesus monkey (Weitzman et al., 1965), the patas monkey *Erythrocebus patas* (Bert and Pegram, 1969), and the primitive nocturnal primate *Galago senegalensis* (Bert et al., 1967b). In the baboon and the vervet monkey *Cercopithecus aethiops,* the lack of continuous delta activity prevents the identification of nonrem stage 4; these two species nevertheless show nonrem substages analogous to human nonrem stages 1, 2, and 3 (Bert and Colomb, 1969; Bert et al., 1967a; Bert and Pegram, 1969).

In many species, rem sleep frequently begins with rhythmic theta activity in cortical leads (Dement, 1967), though in the rhesus monkey the characteristic eye movements of rem sleep begin up to several minutes before the EEG changes from the nonrem to the rem pattern (Weitzman et al., 1965). The sawtooth waves so characteristic of human rem sleep are prominent in the chimpanzee where they also often appear just before or during an eye movement (Freemon et al., 1969). In the chimpanzee, sawtooth waves frequently occur in midbrain reticular formation at the same time as they appear in cortex. Figure 3 presents bursts of theta activity during rem sleep from each of five chimpanzees. In some of the animals the notch on each wave gives the appearance of sawteeth. Weitzman et al. (1965) have reported six per second sawtooth waves in the cortical EEG of the rhesus, but these waveforms have not been identified in other species. Jouvet (1962) in cat and Weitzman et al. (1965) in monkey have recorded rhythmic 6 to 8 cps activity in pontine reticular formation during rem sleep.

Very characteristic of rem sleep in the cat is a continuous rhythmic 5 to 7 cps activity in the hippocampus. This hippocampal theta rhythm occurs in both dorsal and ventral hippocampus, and a similar rhythm can be recorded from pulvinar, periacqueductal gray, medial geniculate nucleus, and limbic midbrain area (Jouvet 1962, 1967; Desiraju et al., 1966). A prominent theta rhythm occurring during rem sleep has been recorded from hippocampus and other limbic areas in rat (Soulairac et al., 1965; Timo-Iaria et al., 1970), rabbit (Khazan and Sawyer, 1964), dog (Shimazono et al., 1960), mole (Van Twyver and Allison 1970a), opossum (Van Twyver and Allison, 1970b), and many other rodent species (Van Twyver, 1969). Both Reite et al. (1965) and Weitzman et al. (1965) specifically noted the absence of hippocampal theta during rem sleep in the rhesus monkey. The chimpanzee and man are discussed in the next chapter. Hippocampal theta rhythm also occurs under certain conditions during wakefulness; however, the rhythm is usually a bit slower in frequency and is usually restricted to the dorsal hippocampus, a structure which has almost disappeared in man. Hippocampal theta occurs in the waking cat during exploration of a new environment (Brown, 1968), during the orienting response (Grastyan et al., 1959, 1966), during learning situations (Adey et al., 1960, 1961, 1962), during voluntary movement (Vanderwolf, 1969; Dalton and Black, 1968; Sainsbury, 1970), during periods when an animal holds itself prepared to make a response (Klemm, 1970), whenever an animal compares new with

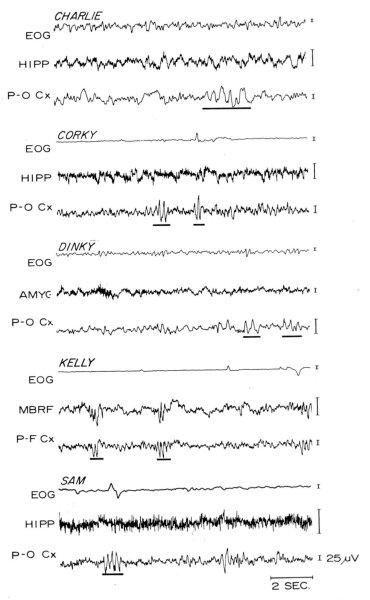

Figure 3. Bursts of theta activity occur in the cortical leads of five chimpanzees during the rem state. In some of these animals a notch on each wave gives the burst the appearance of sawteeth. Similar sawtooth waves occur in human EEG recordings during rem sleep. From Freemon, McNew, and Adey (1969).

remembered information (Pickenhain and Klingberg, 1967), and when the animal focuses its attention on a new, meaningful stimulus (Bennett, 1971). Komisaruk (1970) found hippocampal theta in the rat when and only when the animal was sniffing. The rat's vibrissae, both during waking with hippocampal theta rhythm and during rem sleep, vibrated synchronously with the electrical rhythm recorded from the hippocampus. Hippocampal theta rhythm can be induced by electrical stimulation of the midbrain reticular formation during waking but not during nonrem sleep (Traczyk et al., 1969). A major unanswered question is whether the hippocampal theta rhythm represents an active or an inactive state of the hippocampus. Most workers consider that the hippocampus is physiologically inhibited, perhaps by the reticular system, when occupied by theta activity either during wakefulness or during rem sleep (Parmeggiani, 1967; Rhodes, 1969).

SPONTANEOUS NEURONAL DISCHARGE RATE

Microelectrodes implanted in specific brain areas can record the firing of individual neurons or neuronal processes. Most neurons decrease their firing rate as an animal falls asleep. When the sleeping animal enters rem sleep, most neurons increase their discharge rate to the level of or even higher than the rate during relaxed wakefulness. Podvoll and Goodman (1967) tried to differentiate two types of unit activity response to sleep stage changes. Neurons in brain stem reticular formation and in both specific and nonspecific nuclei of the thalamus showed the highest firing rate during aroused wakefulness and para-doxical sleep with progressively decreasing unit activity as the animal passed through quiet wakefulness, drowsiness, and nonrem sleep. Neurons in caudate nucleus, putamen, hippocampus, amygdala, coch-lear nucleus, and both superior and inferior colliculi showed increases in unit activity associated with arousal and movement and sustained but small increases during rem sleep, but showed much less relationship to behavior state than the reticular and thalamic neurons. Table VII summarizes many studies which seem to show a general relationship of spontaneous unit activity to sleep states. As the animal passes from wakefulness through nonrem sleep to rem sleep, unit activity decreases with the first transition but increases with the second. The interpretation of this generalization is complicated by our lack of knowledge of the physiological meaning of changes in unit activity. Evarts (1969)

TABLE VII

SPONTANEOUS UNIT ACTIVITY DURING SLEEP

Changes from:

Waking to Nonrem Sleep	Nonrem to Rem Sleep	Authors
Pyramidal tract		
decrease	increase	Arduini et al. (1963)
decrease	increase	Evarts (1964)
decrease	increase	Rougeul et al. (1966)
Cerebral cortex, posterior or visual:		
decrease	increase	Evarts (1962)
decrease	increase	Hobson and McCarley (1971a)
decrease	increase	McCarley and Hobson (1970)
decrease	increase	Noda and Adey (1970)
Thalamus		
VPL nucleus:		
decrease	increase	Benoit et al. (1965)
Lateral geniculate body:		
decrease	increase	Benoit (1967)
no change	increase	Mukhametov et al. (1970)
slight decrease	increase	Sakakura (1968)
decrease	increase	Thomas et al. (1968)
Reticular nuclei:		
decrease	increase	Mukhametov et al. (1970)
Midline nucleus:		
decrease	increase	Rougeul et al. (1966)
VL nucleus:		
decrease	increase	Lamarre et al. (1971)
Hippocampus		
decrease	increase	Noda et al. (1969)
no change	decrease	Mink et al. (1967)
Caudate nucleus:		
decrease	increase	Rougeul et al. (1966)
Red nucleus:		
decrease	increase	Gassel et al. (1965)
Midbrain reticular formation:		
decrease	increase	Balzano and Jeannerod (1970)
decrease	increase	Benoit (1964)
no change	increase	Huttenlocher (1961)
decrease	increase	Kasamatsu (1970)
decrease	increase	Manohar et al. (1972)
Pontine reticular formation:		
decrease	no change	Balzano and Jeannerod (1970)
Bulbar reticular formation:		
decrease	increase	Rougeul et al. (1966)
Raphe nucleus:		
decrease	increase	Balzano and Jeannerod (1970)

Nucleus gracilis:		
no change	no change	Belugo and Benoit (1966)
Cochlear nucleus:		
no change	no change	Huttenlocher (1960)
decrease	increase	Winters et al. (1967)
Vestibular nuclei:		
minor changes	minor changes	Bizzi et al. (1964)
Corpus callosum:		
decrease	decrease	Berlucchi (1965)
Purkinje cells:		
decrease	increase	Hobson and McCarley (1970)
no change	increase	Mano (1970)
Amygdala		
increase	decrease	Jacobs and McGinty (1971)

points out that "studies in neuronal activity have been more valuable in indicating what sleep is not than what it is." The review of the literature in sleep unit activity has been eased by Hobson and McCarley's (1971b) annotated bibliography.

One difficulty in interpreting this generalization is that neuronal firing rate averaged over a long period does not give an accurate picture of neuronal activity. Many brain areas show a continuous, unclustered, well-spaced, high frequency discharge during wakefulness, but bursts of increased activity against a relatively silent background during sleep. In nonrem sleep, burst discharges concomitant to sleep spindles in the scalp or cortical EEG characterize some thalamic neurons (Rougeul et al., 1966), neurons of the red nucleus (Gassel et al., 1965), neurons of the raphe nucleus (Balzano and Jeannerod, 1970), and the pyramidal cells of the somatosensory cortex (Arduini et al., 1963) and their axonal processes as recorded from the medullary pyramids (Whitlock et al., 1953; Morrison and Pompeiano, 1965). In rem sleep, a phasic increase in firing rate associated with eye movements and PGO waves occurs in many neurons including those of the pontine reticular formation (Balzano and Jeannerod, 1970), medial and descending vestibular nuclei (Bizzi et al., 1964), raphe nucleus (Balzano and Jeannerod, 1970), mid-brain reticular formation (Huttenlocher 1961; Kasamatsu, 1970), red nucleus (Gassel et al., 1965), lateral geniculate body (Bizzi, 1966; Benoit, 1967; Mukhametov, 1970), and the visual cortex (Calvet et al., 1965; Valleala,

1967; McCarley and Hobson, 1970). The spontaneous rate of fire of Purkinje neurons during rem sleep phasically decreases during eye movements (Marchesi and Strata, 1970). Brief myoclonic jerks of the extremities occurring during rem sleep are sometimes accompanied by a burst of unit activity in somatosensory cortex (Arduini et al., 1963) and the red nucleus (Gassel et al., 1965).

Another difficulty in interpreting unit activity data lies in the fact that many neurons in each brain site differ in their response to sleep stage changes from the majority response summarized in Table VII. The selective bias for large neurons inherent in microelectrode work means that the activity of the "average" neuron of the table may not even be typical of the majority of neurons as defined histologically. Even if the "average" neuron follows the general rule of decreasing activity in nonrem and increasing activity in rem, many neurons are exceptions to this generalization. In the cerebral cortex, neurons which discharge at a high rate during wakefulness show the typical pattern, decreasing their activity during nonrem and increasing it during rem sleep; however, those neurons which discharge at a slow rate during wakefulness increase their firing rate as the animal falls into nonrem sleep (Creutzfield and Jung, 1961) and increase their activity still more during the transition from nonrem to rem sleep (Hobson and McCarley, 1971a). Evarts (1962) found that the critical discharge frequency during wakefulness was about 8 per second; units firing above this rate decreased, and those firing below this rate increased as the animal fell asleep. Evarts (1965) postulated that the larger neocortical pyramidal neurons increased rate, and the smaller ones decreased rate during transition from waking to nonrem sleep.

Since the hypothalamus contains many cell types related to many neurovegetative functions, it is not surprising to find many different changes in firing patterns during sleep. Parmeggiani and Franzini (1970, 1971) found that neurons of the anterior and dorsal hypothalamus usually decreased their rates of discharge in nonrem sleep and further decreased their activity in rem sleep, while lateral hypothalamic units showed an increase in rate during transition to rem sleep except for the tuberal division of the lateral hypothalamus which showed a decrease during rem sleep. Unit activity of the fornix, mammillary body, and mammillothalamic tract decreased their activity during nonrem sleep, especially late in a nonrem period, but showed an increased discharge rate during rem sleep. These results occurred at every environmental temperature except, of course, those which blocked the appearance of the rem state. Vincent et al. (1967) found very few units in the premammillary region; those which they encountered did not change firing rate with change in sleep stages. In the dorsal portion of the ventromedian complex, neurons decreased firing rate during nonrem and increased during rem. Oomura and his co-workers (1969) reported that cells in the ventromedial nucleus had a higher discharge rate in nonrem sleep than in either rem sleep or waking. Findlay and Hayward (1969) performed one of the most thorough studies of hypothalamic unit activity during sleep, concluding that "hypothalamic cells do not behave as a homogeneous population in relation to changes in the state of arousal." Twenty-five of the thirty-two cells which could be followed through both stages of sleep showed higher rates during rem sleep than during wakefulness, but six cells showed decreased activity, and two of these, one in lateral and one in dorsomedial hypothalamus, showed complete cessation of activity during rem sleep. Lincoln (1969) found that about half of the hypothalamic units he recorded had the same activity in both sleep states; about a quarter fired faster in rem than in nonrem sleep, and about a quarter had a higher discharge rate in nonrem than in rem sleep. He also found that some hypothalamic but no cortical neurons had an unusual firing pattern only during the two-minute transition period as the animal entered rem sleep.

In summary, unit activity data is hard to correlate with other aspects of sleep research since we do not know the meaning behind changes in neuronal discharge rates. The generalization that the majority of neurons during rem increase and nonrem decrease their firing rates holds for most brain areas. Certain regions are exceptions to this rule including dorsal hippocampus (Mink et al., 1967), certain hypothalamic regions, and basolateral amygdala (Jacobs and McGinty, 1971). Perhaps more significant than discharge rate is discharge pattern. The rapid but well-spaced and unclustered discharge pattern of wakefulness changes during sleep to a pattern of neuronal discharge in bursts, associated with cortical spindles during nonrem sleep and with PGO spikes and eye movements during rem sleep. Unit activity research has definitely shown that any simplistic concepts relating sleep to a period of neuronal standstill must be discarded.

LOCALIZATION OF THE SLEEP MECHANISM

In the attempt to delineate the neural structures involved in the production of nonrem and rem sleep, investigators have used the traditional methods of electrical stimulation and lesion production. In addition, pharmacologic interference with the synthesis of neurotransmitter substances can show that certain types of neurons participate in sleep generation.

Electrical stimulation can induce nonrem sleep. Cats, when stimulated in the following brain regions, usually curl up and go to sleep within a minute or two: medial thalamus (Hess, 1956), basal forebrain (Sterman and Clemente, 1962), raphe nucleus of the midbrain (Kostowski et al., 1969), caudate nucleus, mammillary body (Parmeggiani, 1962), and cerebral neocortex (Penaloza-Rojas et al, 1964). Since cats tend to fall asleep quite readily in the laboratory situation, the specificity of this stimulation remains open to question. Negative points (those brain locations where electrical stimulation is not followed by sleep) in these studies may be related to the production of pain, fear, uneasiness, or some other emotional interference with sleep. Roelofs et al. (1963), using sham stimulation as a control, found decreased latencies to sleep following electrical stimulation of cerebellum, hippocampus, amygdala, and neocortex. Pompeiano and Swett (1962) actually produced sleep by low rate stimulation of peripheral nerves. In all of these stimulation studies, the parameters of stimulation are at least as important as the site. Sleep follows low voltage stimulation at low stimulation rates, about 4 to 10 times per second. Higher voltage and/or higher stimulation rates can produce arousal. Of course, many things can influence the act of falling asleep. There exists evidence in the cat (Drucker-Colin et al., 1970) and rabbit (Monnier et al., 1963) that a circulating substance helps induce sleep. On the other hand, human Siamese twins sharing the same circulation can sleep independently of one another (Brown, 1959). Several workers have reported that stimulation of certain brain sites in the cat including pontine and midbrain reticular formation, hypothalamus, and hippocampus can produce rem sleep, but only when the stimulation occurs during nonrem sleep (Rossi et al., 1961; Cadilhac et al., 1963; Parmeggiani and Zanocco, 1963; Monti, 1970; Frederickson and Hobson, 1970). Kripke et al. (1966) could not confirm this phenomenon in the monkey and suggested that the feline results had been related to the fact that a cat in nonrem sleep is about to enter rem sleep regardless of electrical stimulation. Electrical stimulation producing arousal will be discussed in Chapter 6.

While certain brain lesions can affect sleep stage percentages, other lesions abolish only one aspect of a sleep stage, such as the eye movements of rem sleep, without affecting the other elements of that stage. Some of the difficulties of this type of research have been emphasized by McGinty (1969). He found that rats went through three different stages following lesions of posterior hypothalamus and subthalamic area. For a few hours after the lesion, the animals showed hyperactivity with sleeplessness. The next few days the animals were somnolent with slow waves and spindles in the EEG. Recovery from this period of somnolence produced an animal which actually slept less than normal animals. The general result of localized brain lesions, however, is summarized in Table VIII. Despite fairly good phylogenetic stability of the result of these lesions, no clear picture of sleep control mechanisms emerges.

Transection of the brain stem at different levels allows separation of the sleep behavior of those portions of the nervous system rostral to the cut from the behavior of the nervous system caudal to the lesion (Bremer, 1935; Moruzzi 1964). Section at the junction of the midbrain and cerebrum produces constant slow waves and spindles in the cerebrum. The episodes of hypotonia which occur in this preparation may be related to rem-like behavior of the brain stem caudal to the transection (Jouvet, 1962). Section of the brain stem between midbrain and pons also produces slow waves and spindles in the cortical EEG; however, this slow activity can be disrupted and replaced by low voltage, fast frequency activity following electrical stimulation of the midbrain reticular formation or following olfactory stimuli such as meat, but not visual stimuli such as flashing lights (Arduini and Moruzzi, 1953; Villablanca, 1965). Similar episodes of hypotonia occur in this preparation. A transection through the pons just rostral to the trigeminal nucleus produces a preparation whose afferent and efferent connections are the same, but whose behavior is totally

TABLE VIII

THE EFFECT OF BRAIN LESIONS UPON SLEEP PATTERNS

Lesion	Result	Species	Reference
Posterior hypothalamus	Somnolence: slow waves and spindles in EEG	rat cat monkey	Nauta (1946); McGinty (1969) Nakamura and Ohye (1964) Ranson (1939); Kennard (1943)
Midbrain reticular formation	Coma; slow waves and spindles in EEG	cat monkey man	Lindsley et al. (1950) French and Magoun (1952) French (1952); Mason-Browne (1956)
Hippocampal complex	Frequent awakenings from nonrem sleep; no change in rem sleep	cat	Kim et al. (1971)
Fastigial nucleus of cerebellum	Decreased nonrem sleep; no change in rem sleep	cat	Giannazzo et al. (1968)
Pontine reticular formation	Rem sleep abolished	cat	Carli and Zanchetti (1965)
Preoptic basal forebrain	Insomnia	cat	McGinty and Sterman (1968)
Raphe nuclei of pons	Insomnia	cat	Jouvet (1969, 1972)
Vestibular nuclei	Abolishes the eye movements and other phasic elements of rem sleep but not the state itself	cat man (?)	Morrison and Pompeiano (1970) Appenzeller and Fischer (1968)
Caudal locus coeruleus	Abolishes hypotonia but not other aspects of rem sleep	cat	Jouvet and Delorme (1965)
Septal nucleus	Abolishes hippocampal theta rhythm but not other aspects of rem sleep	rat cat	Brugge (1965) Parmeggiani and Zanocco (1963)
Thalamus	Abolishes spindles in cortical EEG but does not change sleep stage amounts	cat man	Angeleri et al. (1969) Jurko and Andy (1965)

different than the prepontine sectioned animal. The neocortex shows
low voltage, fast frequency activity most of the time (Batini et al.,
1959; Slosarska and Zernicki, 1969). The animal sometimes follows a
vertically moving object with his eyes (King and Marchiafava, 1963).
Lateral eye movements do not occur because the abducens nucleus
is below the transection. Brain stem transection between pons and
medulla produces similar behavior in the rostral preparation and
erases the episodes of hypotonia triggered by the nervous system
caudal to previous transections. These results suggest that neural elements in the pons participate in the generation of wakefulness and
possibly of rem sleep. Carli and Zanchett (1965) suggested that the
nucleus reticularis pontis oralis was this "rem sleep center," while
Jouvet (1969, 1972) has implicated the pontine portion of the locus
coeruleus.

Pharmacologic interference with sleep patterns helps identify the
type of neurotransmitter substance involved in the initiation or maintenance of each type of sleep. Serotonin neurons play a part in the
neural mechanism which initiates nonrem sleep (Jouvet, 1968, 1969,
1972). Lesions which include the serotonin containing cells of the
raphe nuclei and pharmacologic techniques which block serotonin
synthesis cause insomnia (Jouvet et al., 1966; Mouret et al., 1967;
Kostowski et al., 1968; Torda, 1969; Koella, 1969). In these two
situations, if a small dose of the serotonin precursor, 5-hydroxytrypto-
phan is given, the animal rapidly falls to nonrem sleep (Pujol et al.,
1971). Rem sleep appears in these preparations only after nonrem
sleep has returned to a certain level. This effect occurs in the cat, rat,
rabbit, and monkey (Florio et al., 1968; Weitzman et al., 1968). In
man, on the other hand, a block in serotonin synthesis decreases rem
but not nonrem sleep (Wyatt et al., 1969a) and the administration of
serotonin precursors induces rem sleep (Oswald et al., 1966; Wyatt
et al., 1971c).

A cholinergic system may also participate in the induction of sleep.
Application of acetyl choline anywhere along the median forebrain
bundle from the orbital frontal cortex to the midbrain reticular formation induces sleep (Hernandez-Peon et al., 1967; Mazzuchelli-
O'Flaherty et al., 1967). Lesions in the median forebrain bundle block
the sleep response of acetyl choline applied rostral to the lesion
(Hernandez-Peon et al., 1963). The injection of atropine into the

median forebrain bundle produces a reversible block of this descending sleep inducing system (Velluti and Hernandez-Peon, 1963). Acetylcholine also produces sleep when applied to the bulbar but not the pontine reticular formation (Cordeau et al., 1963). One might expect that blocking brain synthesis of acteylcholine would produce insomnia; actually intrathecal injection of hemicholinium, which inhibits acetylcholine formation, markedly inhibits only rem sleep even at small doses (Hazra, 1970; Domino and Stawiski, 1971). Systemic administration of atropine can produce slow waves in the neocortex even in the waking cat (Wikler, 1952). Indirect evidence suggests that neural elements which include noradrenergic neurons participate in the induction of rem sleep (reviewed by Hartmann, 1970).

Mandell and his co-workers (1969) have suggested that the degree of implication of serotonin, acetylcholine, and norepinephrine in sleep control mechanisms is proportional to the power of the experimental methods available to examine the function of that neurotransmitter substance. They compare our present understanding of the sleep mechanism to the drunk looking for his keys under the street lamp though he dropped them half a block away. Both the drunk and the pharmacologist have chosen their areas of investigation because that is where the light is. Mandell et al. (1969) have presented evidence that neurotransmitters such as glycine, gamma-amino butyrate, and many others play just as important a role in controlling sleep as does serotonin.

MENTAL ACTIVITY DURING ANIMAL SLEEP

I used to have a dog. Actually it was the neighbor's dog, but we were in a "no-pet" apartment building, and the landlord was always stomping up to the Bonjeans' apartment to look for this dog, and the Bonjeans would hide Valentine in our apartment. Especially when he was a puppy, he had the habit of moaning in his sleep. One time in particular comes to mind. Valentine was sleeping on the rug in the middle of the living room. He started sleeping on his side but when I noticed his low moans begin he had rolled onto his back with his four paws in the air. As he moaned his paws twitched, and beneath his half-closed lids I could see his eyes moving conjugately back and forth. The low moans changed into pitiful howls so loud that my wife called down from upstairs, "What are you doing to that dog?"

"Shuddup! I'm studying his sleep," I shouted back, but neither of these cries awakened him. Finally the howling grew so plaintive that my wife came downstairs in a huff and shook the dog awake, commenting, "Can't you see he is in pain?" The awakened puppy looked around in a bewildered manner, then lay back down on his side and went back to sleep without eye movements. I think I need a polygraph in my home.

Everyone has had experiences with sleeping animals similar to my experience with Valentine. Most people who have extensive contact with animals accept that animals have mental experiences during their sleep. Scientists, especially scientists working with human subjects, have emphasized man's unique mental attributes and have denied that animals experience emotions during rem sleep. Animals with extensive lesions that interrupt waking activities and presumably waking mentation, may continue to show the eye movements and muscular twitches of rem sleep. In an unpublished thesis, Vaughn (1963) reported that monkeys, trained to press a button during wakefulness when they saw visual images, suddenly began pressing the button during sleep. These monkeys were not monitored polygraphically so that Vaughn was unable to correlate sleep stage with this suggested occurrence of visual imagery during sleep (related by Snyder, 1967). Jouvet (1969, 1972) reported that lesions which included caudal portions of the locus coeruleus produced cats which had the EEG and eye movements of rem sleep but lacked the inhibition of muscle activity. These cats hissed and scratched as though they were reacting to imaginary images.

In summary, there is little scientific, but much anecdotal evidence that animals experience ongoing mental activity during sleep. Jack London (1903) described the sleep mentation of the dog, Buck, and suggested that the mental activity included elements from previous generations, a sort of Jungian collective unconscious of dogs:

> Best of all, perhaps, he loved to lie near the fire, hind legs crouched under him, forelegs stretched out in front, head raised, and eyes blinking dreamily at the flames. Sometimes he thought of Judge Miller's big house in the sun-kissed Santa Clara valley, and of the cement swimming tank, and Ysabel, the Mexican hairless, and Toots, the Japanese pug; but oftener he remembered the man in the red sweater, the death of Curly, the great fight with Spitz, and the good things he had eaten or would like

to eat. Far more potent were the memories of his heredity that gave things he had never seen before a seeming familiarity; the instincts (which were but the memories of his ancestors become habits) which had lapsed in later days, and still later, in him, quickened and became alive again.

Sometimes as he crouched there, blinking dreamily at the flames, it seemed that the flames were of another fire, and that as he crouched by this other fire he saw another and different man from the half-breed cook before him. This other man was shorter of leg and longer of arm, with muscles that were stringy and knotty rather than rounded and swelling. The hair of this man was long and matted, and his head slanted back under it from the eyes. He uttered strange sounds, and seemed very much afraid of the darkness, into which he peered continually, clutching in his hand, which hung midway between knee and foot, a stick with a heavy stone made fast to the end.

And beyond the fire, in the circling darkness, Buck could see many gleaming coals, two by two, always two by two, which he knew to be the eyes of great beasts of prey. And he could hear the crashing of their bodies through the undergrowth, and the noises they made in the night. And dreaming there by the Yukon bank, with lazy eyes blinking at the fire, these sounds and sights of another world would make the hair to rise along his back and stand on end across his shoulders and up to his neck, till he whimpered low and suppressedly, or growled softly, and the half-breed cook shouted at him, "Hey, you Buck, wake up!" Whereupon the other world would vanish and the real world would come into his eyes, and he would get up and yawn and stretch as though he had been asleep. [Slightly abridged from Jack London's *Call of the Wild,* 1903]

OTHER ASPECTS OF FELINE REM SLEEP

Eye movements during rem sleep in cat are conjugate, come in bursts or singly. These movements continue in the decorticate animal (Jouvet, 1962) but are abolished by brain stem lesions which include the medial and inferior vestibular nuclei (Pompeiano and Morrison, 1965). The pupil remains constricted during rem as during nonrem sleep but shows a slight dilatation concomitant with each eye movement (Berlucchi et al., 1964). Lesions of the medial and inferior vestibular nuclei abolish the slight pupillary dilatation and the brief increases in heart rate which accompany the eye movements of rem sleep (Morrison and Pompeiano, 1970).

PGO waves are distinctive, high amplitude, sharp waves occurring in several brain sites during rem sleep usually associated with an eye movement (Brooks and Bizzi, 1963). The term is derived from three brain locations where this activity can be recorded: pontine reticular formation, lateral geniculate body, and occipital cortex. Similar waveforms occur in the brain stem nuclei which supply the extraocular muscles. PGO waves usually occur immediately prior to each eye movement. Costin and Hafeman (1970) observed that a PGO wave in the lateral geniculate body preceeded every eye movement while PGO waves in the oculomotor nucleus only occurred associated with an eye movement which required contraction of a muscle supplied by that nucleus. Electrical stimulation of the pontine reticular formation during rem but not during nonrem sleep produces PGO waves in both lateral geniculate bodies while stimulation in the lateral geniculate body causes no change in the spontaneous electrical activity of the pons or the other lateral geniculate nucleus (Bizzi and Brooks, 1963; Malcolm et al., 1970). Enucleation of the eye has no immediate effect on PGO wave generation, but following optic nerve and tract degeneration these waveforms disappear from lateral geniculate nucleus but not from pons (Brooks, 1967). These findings suggest that PGO waves are triggered in the pontine reticular formation and proceed to the cranial nerve nuclei which supply extraocular muscles and to the lateral geniculate body and the occipital cortex. Hobson et al. (1969) recorded PGO waves from occipital cortex of animals with lesions in both lateral geniculate bodies and postulated the existence of an extrageniculate pathway which transmitted PGO activity from pons to occipital cortex. PGO waves can occasionally be recorded during wakefulness associated with waking eye movements (Brooks, 1968), but unlike the PGO waves of rem sleep the amplitude of these waveforms depends upon retinal illumination (Brooks and Gershon, 1971). The PGO wave of rem sleep usually precedes the eye movement; the PGO wave of wakefulness usually follows the eye movement (Jeannerod and Sakai, 1970). The PGO wave studies discussed up until now have all been performed in the cat. Monophasic waves have also been recorded from pons and from the lateral geniculate nucleus of the monkey associated with waking eye movements (Cohen and Feldman, 1968). As illustrated in the next chapter, sharp waves occur in human and in chimpanzee midbrain reticular formation during rem sleep but the relationship of these sharp potentials to feline PGO waves remains unknown.

A marked decrease in the monosynaptic deep tendon reflexes occurs during rem sleep, presumably due to a descending inhibitory pathway directly to the alpha motor neurons (Pompeiano, 1969). Panting and shivering disappear during rem sleep regardless of the environmental temperature and Parmeggiani and Rabini (1970) have postulated that the cat becomes poikilothermic during the rem state. Since rem deprivation is frequently utilized to study neurochemical changes during the rem state, biochemical sleep studies will be discussed in the chapter on sleep deprivation.

Chapter 4

COMPARISON OF HUMAN AND CHIMPANZEE SLEEP

As a rule the early ancestors of man, including *Ramapithecus* and subsequent species, probably used the trees to sleep in. When trees were not available, they chose places where predators could not follow, perhaps spending their nights on the ledges of cliffs facing the cliff wall as some baboons do in the twentieth century. During the day they ventured into grassy savannas and semiarid regions, exploiting every available source of food.

PFEIFFER, *The Emergence of Man*

SLEEP OF CHIMPANZEE

SINCE the chimpanzee is man's closest evolutionary relative, study of his sleep in the laboratory may amplify our knowledge of human sleep and its relationships to sleep of the cat, rat, and other mammals. Unlike these latter animals, the chimpanzee dislikes flexible cables connecting his head to a fixed point, and the unrestrained chimp will rip the cables from their fixtures. This problem complicates the monitoring of brain electrophysiologic signals. Early studies recorded cerebral activity and other physiologic varibles by restraining the chimp in a chair in such a manner that he could not reach the monitoring cables.

The first modern physiologic studies of the sleep of chimpanzee were by W.R. Adey, J.M. Rhodes, and their colleagues at the Space Biology Laboratory of the Brain Research Institute at the University of California, Los Angeles (Adey et al., 1963; Rhodes et al., 1963, 1964). These workers found that the cortical electrical activity during sleep as recorded by screw electrodes in the skull was quite similar to the scalp EEG in man. They stated that it was possible to differentiate chimpanzee sleep into stages analogous to human sleep including nonrem sleep's four substages, but they gave no specific figures, probably because of the fragmented and obviously abnormal sleep

51

pattern of the restrained animal. Depth electrode recordings revealed variable and complex hippocampal and amygdala activity during sleep. W.H. Rickles (1965) studied the restrained chimpanzee at the Aeromedical Research Laboratory, Holloman Air Force Base, New Mexico. He also found cortical EEG during chimp sleep to be similar to human scalp recordings. The animals frequently strained against their restraints, especially in the first part of the night, and when they did fall asleep they demonstrated frequent sleep stage changes and frequent awakenings. In a total of twelve nights recorded from four animals, five were associated with either no rem sleep or a total absence of nonrem stage 4. By eliminating these nights, Rickels obtained sleep stage values of 13.9 percent awake time, 31.3 percent stage 1, 37.9 percent stage 2, 6.0 percent stage 3, 3.6 percent stage 4, and 5.6 percent stage rem on the relatively undisturbed nights. Rickels concluded that this low amount of rem and slow wave sleep was probably because "the animals were doubtlessly very uncomfortable and in an unnatural sleeping position." Rickels also found that respiratory rate increased, and amplitude of chest excursion with each breath decreased as the animal entered the rem stage. Heart rate increased during rem sleep periods, but the electromyogram of the chin and back showed no differences between rem and nonrem stages though there was a marked drop of muscle tension as the animal passed from wakefulness to sleep.

Telemetry technique allows physiologic monitoring of the unrestrained chimpanzee. I was fortunate to be a research fellow at the Space Biology Laboratory during the period when engineering advances in telemetry were beginning to bear fruit. Figure 4 shows an unrestrained chimpanzee about to be placed in his home cage for all-night recording. The records of five animals were evaluated for depth activity, and the records of two animals were formally scored for sleep stages. Visual analysis of all-night records revealed a striking similarity between chimpanzee cortical activity during sleep as sampled by electrodes screwed into the skull and human cortical activity during sleep as sampled by electrodes applied to the scalp. Most animals showed a definite rhythm about 8 to 10 cps when resting with eyes closed. As the animals became drowsy, this rhythm disappeared. Occasional vertex sharp waves appeared at this time. The posterior neck muscle EMG activity decreased. Spindles and K-complexes appeared but were gradually replaced by 1 to 2 cps slow waves. The latter activity progressed until essentially continuous slow activity occupied cortex for several minutes. This progression was never direct but was interrupted by awakenings and shifts among

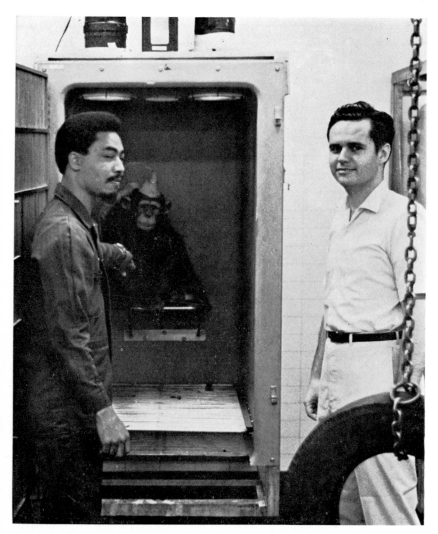

Figure 4. Charlie is being put to bed. The chimpanzee wears a telemetry pack strapped to his back and connected by cable to his permanent electrode plug. The animal's behavior is observed throughout the night by means of the television camera atop the cage.

the nonrem substages. Only after two or three hours of this activity did the first rem period appear. A burst of 3 to 5 cps activity often heralded the change in EEG to a low voltage activity with intermixed theta and saw-tooth waves. Eye movements usually began after about a minute of the EEG change.

Chimpanzee polygraphic records were so similar to those of man that the records could be scored by the Rechtschaffen and Kales (1968) modification of the Dement and Kleitman (1957) scoring rules for human sleep stages. The EMG showed a decrease in amplitude during transition from wakefulness to sleep but was not helpful in differentiating rem from nonrem sleep. All scoring was done on the basis of the cortical EEG channels and the electro-oculogram without reference to the electrical activity of subcortical structures. The records from seven consecutive nights from two of our animals were scored for sleep stages strictly by these criteria. Since the first night of sleep in the chimpanzee contains more time awake and less time in stage rem than later nights (McNew, Howe, and Adey, 1971), analysis was restricted to nights two through seven in order to be sure that a "first night effect" did not muddy the description of sleep patterns in normal juvenile chimpanzee.

During the twelve hours between lights out at 1900 and lights on at 0700, the two animals spent an average of 652.4 minutes asleep and 62.2 minutes awake. An average of 5.4 minutes per night was obscured by artifact. Of the time sleep, 8 percent was stage 1, 44 percent stage 2, 15 percent stage 3, 10 percent stage 4, and 23 percent stage rem (Freemon et al., 1971). The majority of stage 2 and much of stage rem occurred during the latter portions of the sleeping period while almost all of stage 4 took place before 0100. Figure 5 gives the graphed sleep pattern from each animal for each night. From these graphs one can calculate the cycle length; that is, the length of time from the beginning of one rem period to the beginning of the next rem period. For nights two through seven, the sleep cycle was 86.1 minutes in length in the animal Kelly and 85.2 minutes in length in Corky. About 6 to 8 cycles occurred per night.

The sleep of unrestrained chimpanzees has also been studied at the chimpanzee colony at Holloman Air Force Base, New Mexico. Bert, Kripke, and Rhodes (1970) found that these adult animals spent only 15 percent of their sleeping time in the rem state. The total

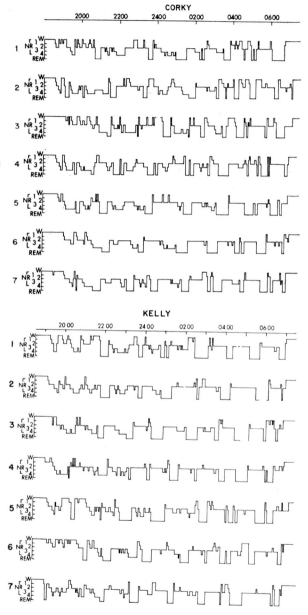

Figure 5. Sleep patterns from seven consecutive nights from two chimpanzees. Most of nonrem stages 3 and 4 occur early in the night. From Freemon, Mc-New, and Adey (1971).

sleep time was less in the chimpanzees studied by Bert and his co-workers than in our animals; the stage 4 sleep percentage was identical in the two studies. Several drug, scoring, and environmental differences could account for this difference in rem percentage, 15 versus 23, but we think it most likely that the maturity of the animals is the major factor. The Holloman animals were sexually mature, weighing 39 to 52 kilograms. Our animals were 4 years old, were sexually immature, and weighed about 14 kilograms. Probably the chimpanzee, like man, rat, cat, and guinea pig shows decreasing rem percentage and sleep time during development (Jouvet-Mounier et al., 1970; Gramsbergen et al., 1970; Rhodes et al., 1971).

In addition to describing sleep stages in the chimpanzee, my colleagues and I evaluated depth electrical activity by visual analysis (Freemon et al., 1969). Most subcortical sites, including head of caudate nucleus and midbrain reticular formation, showed low voltage, fast frequency activity during rem periods and high voltage, slow frequency activity during nonrem sleep. The amygdala showed a number of different types of electrical activity. The usual appearance of amygdaloid leads during sleep was a low voltage fast frequency activity without the polyphasic or saw-tooth activity typical of cortex during rem periods. At other times during rem sleep the amygdala showed 2 to 3 cps low voltage rhythmic activity or 6 to 8 cps higher amplitude activity, particularly prominent in the animal Corky. In two animals, bursts of 21 to 24 cps high amplitude activity occurred in some rem periods but not others (Fig. 6). When the amygdaloid bursts began in these two animals when awake, the chimpanzee usually showed obvious excitement or fear and sometimes they howled loudly. Anterior hippocampus showed several types of electrical activity during sleep. As shown in Figure 7, low voltage, fast frequency activity could occur in hippocampus during rem sleep, or wakefulness, a 2 to 3 cps activity could occur in either type of sleep, and 4 to 6 cps irregular monophasic high amplitude sharp waves could occur in either nonrem sleep or wakefulness. All the examples of Figure 7 are taken from a single animal on a single night; other animals showed slow activity more clearly; for example, see Charlie's record in Figure 3. Anterior hippocampus also showed a characteristic wave consisting of a slight upward potential, a deep downward sharp wave, and then another upward potential, as shown in Figure 8. These occurred more

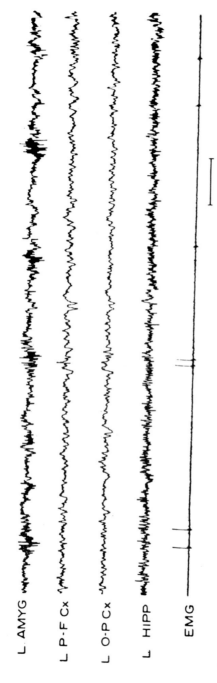

Figure 6. Bursts of 23 to 25 cps activity occur in amygdala in some chimpanzees during rem sleep. These bursts occur less frequently during nonrem and only occur during waking when the animal is excited. From Freemon, McNew, and Adey (1969).

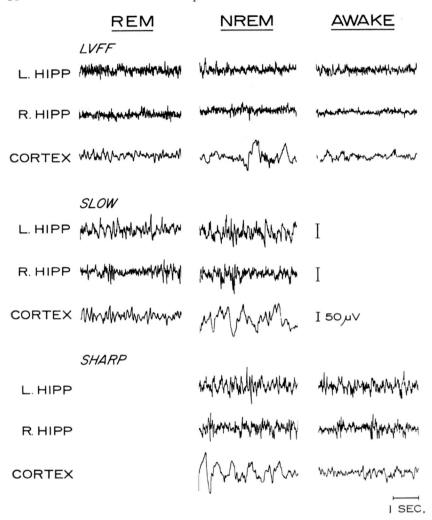

Figure 7. The chimpanzee hippocampus shows several different types of activity during sleep and waking. From Freemon, McNew, and Adey (1969).

frequently in Stage 2 than in Stage 4 and were extremely rare in rem sleep. When the waves were bilateral they were often associated with a K-complex in cortex, but the majority of these waveforms were unilateral, and most K-complexes were unassociated with any change in hippocampal activity.

Another portion of the study compared the first and the last rem

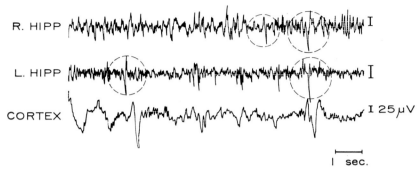

R. HIPP

L. HIPP

CORTEX

I 25 μV

I sec.

Figure 8. A characteristic triphasic waveform (circled) occurs in chimpanzee hippocampus during nonrem sleep. From Freemon, McNew, and Adey (1969).

periods (Freemon et al., 1970). Records from sixteen nights of sleep in four juvenile chimpanzees were randomly selected from the larger study. For the purpose of this analysis, the first rem period was defined as the first occurrence of rem sleep greater than ten minutes in duration occurring after lights out at 1900, and the last period as the last portion of the record with at least ten minutes of continuous rem activity and with the period terminating before lights on at 0700. The electrical activity of cortex and subcortical structures showed no marked differences between first and last rem periods. The only visible difference in the EEG records was the greater apparent frequency of bursts of saw-tooth waves in later rem. We attempted to quantify this apparent difference between early and late rem by counting bursts of saw-tooth waves in cortical channels. We counted each burst of three or more monophasic indented waves whose basic frequency was 3 to 6 cps. This analysis revealed saw-tooth wave bursts to be more frequent in late than in early rem periods, averaging 8.9 per period or 0.37 per minute in late rem and only 4.5 bursts per period or 0.24 per minute in early rem periods. Electro-oculogram activity gave us the definite impression that eye movements occurred more frequently and were of greater amplitude in late than in early rem periods. Eye movements were so frequent that quantification of this difference was not feasible. Body movements, however, proved amenable to quantification, being identified by EMG activity and by direct observation. Counting of these movements showed 2.4 body movements per period or 0.10 per minute during late rem, but only 1.0 per period or 0.053 per minute in early rem periods. The types of movements which made up this difference were mainly nodding or jerking of the head and slight twisting or rolling movements of the body. The duration of the last rem period was longer than the first, 24.3 to 19.0 minutes. If one restricted analysis to only those rem periods which did not terminate with arousal but ended with an uninterrupted transition to nonrem sleep, this difference became greater, 27.7 to 19.7 minutes. All of these results are statistically significant.

DEPTH RECORDINGS DURING SLEEP IN MAN

The delineation of normal electrical activity from subcortical sites of the human brain during sleep is important in order to help compare human sleep to the sleep of experimental animals and in order to better understand the sleep neurophysiology of our own species. The implantation of depth electrodes is not performed in normal man, and attempts to describe normal human depth electrical activity must be extrapolated from the activity recorded from abnormal brains during diagnostic and therapeutic studies of patients.

I encountered a patient with electrodes in hypothalamus and midbrain in an unusual way. While I was waiting to see patients in the neurologic clinic at the Shands Teaching Hospital of the University of Florida, my colleague, Dr. B.J. Wilder, came to me with a skull x-ray showing depth electrodes in unusual locations (Fig. 9). I abandoned the clinic and immediately arranged with H. W. Agnew, Jr., and the neurosurgeons in charge of the patient, and, of course, with the patient himself to study his sleep patterns that very night. The

TABLE IX

FIRST AND LAST REM PERIODS

	CHIMPANZEE		MAN	
	First Rem Period	Last Rem Period	First Rem Period	Last Rem Period
Duration	short	long	short	long
Eye movements	few	many	few	many
Saw-tooth waves	few	many	not compared	not compared
Body movements	few	many	few	many
Rem mentation	?	?	indistinct	vivid

Adapted from Freemon, McNew, and Adey, *Folia Primatologia, 13*:144-149, 1970. Data for man taken from Dement and Kleitman (1957), Goodenough et al. (1965), and Verdone (1965).

patient was a thirty-two-year-old orange grove worker who had had psychomotor seizures since age twelve, probably due to perinatal trauma or anoxia. Because the seizures became intractable to medication, the patient was evaluated for possible temporal lobectomy. Electroencephalograms suggested a persistent right temporal focus. Bilateral carotid arteriograms and pneumoencephalogram were normal. For better definition of the epileptic focus, deep electrodes were placed by the free hand method on March 17, 1967. On the fifth night after placement, the patient slept all night with the electrical activity of cortical and deep structures monitored and with eye movements recorded between electrodes attached to the inferior outer canthus of the left eye and the superior outer canthus of the right eye. The subcortical recordings were obtained from bipolar electrodes with the recording tips one centimeter apart along two separate neurosurgical tracts. By reference to the patient's skull x-rays with electrodes in place (Fig. 9) and to his previous pneumoencephalogram, we placed the same electrodes into cadaver brains which were then sectioned. Though exact localization is impossible due to variations in brain size, it is quite likely that recordings were obtained from the right caudate nucleus along one neurosurgical tract and from midbrain reticular formation and right posterior hypothalamus along the other. Other sites were recorded, but localization is less sure. A bipolar electrode with recording tips one centimeter apart overlay the dura mater in the right parietal cortical area.

During the analysis of the tracings we purposely disregarded any wave forms which had an epileptiform appearance. When the patient was awake and resting, the record showed low voltage, fast frequency activity in all leads. Within 30 minutes of retiring he passed into nonrem stage 4 sleep characterized by high amplitude delta waves beginning simultaneously in cortex, caudate nucleus, and midbrain tegmentum with low voltage, fast frequency activity in posterior hypothalamus. The patient experienced one period of rem sleep early in the night. This stage was accompanied by few rapid eye movements, low voltage fast activity in cortex, caudate, and midbrain with 3 cps rhythmic activity in posterior hypothalamus. Beginning about 0300 the patient experienced lengthy episodes of rem sleep with frequent eye movements, low voltage activity in all leads including hypothalamus, and occasional distinct potentials in midbrain tegmentum.

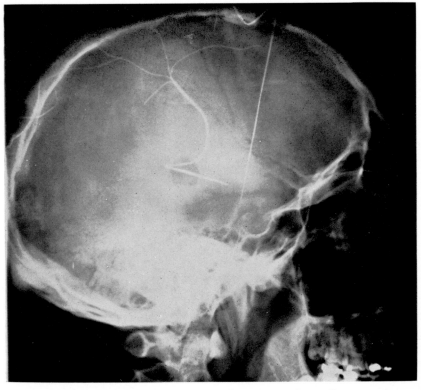

Figure 9. Skull x-ray shows depth electrodes in place. From Freemon, Agnew, and Wilder (1970).

These sharp potentials did not occur in the first rem period. The potentials occurred singly or in bursts of about 3 cps frequency; most often these sharp midbrain waves were either simultaneous with eye movements or immediately preceded them. Figure 10 summarizes these results.

Dr. Richard D. Walter allowed me to examine the all-night depth EEG recordings collected over a period of years by a large number of investigators at UCLA, including L.F. Chapman, P.H. Crandall, C.H. Markham, R.W. Rand, W.H. Rickels, Jr., and R.D. Walter. A total of twelve all-night depth electrode recordings from eight patients were available for analysis. Cases 1 through 5 were temporal lobe epileptics; case 6 was a suspected temporal lobe epileptic who later turned out to have temporal lobe seizures secondary to a brain tumor;

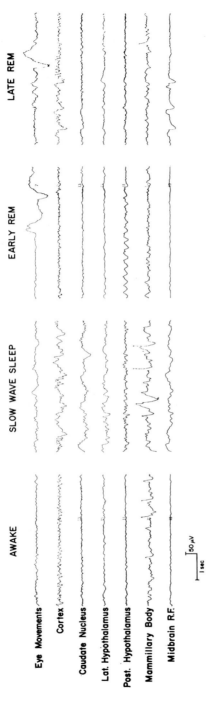

Figure 10. Electrical activity of depth structures in an epileptic patient. Rhythmic theta activity occupies posterior hypothalamus in early rem periods.

cases 7 and 8 were chronic schizophrenics. The sleep of these patients was disturbed with long periods of wakefulness in some cases. Nevertheless, all patients save one had easily recognizable nonrem stage 4 early in the record. Since the patients had frequent periods of wakefulness that might masquerade as a rem period, only unequivocal rem sleep was accepted for analysis. No rem periods of sufficient length and clarity could be identified in three patients, but in the others rem sleep periods occurred frequently, particularly in the early morning hours. Extensive analysis of stage two was not possible because much of the record in the temporal lobe patients was occupied by epileptiform activity and because considerable variation in subcortical waveforms from individual to individual and from period to period in the same individual made generalization difficult. Usually, but not always, the 12 to 15 cps spindle bursts in cortex were accompanied by similar waves in thalamus and in posterior hippocampal complex. In general, however, most subcortical sites remained quite flat throughout stage 2 sleep.

Observations on amygdala and uncus are not included in the rem and stage 4 sleep periods described below because of the independence of the activity of these structures from staging based on cortical and eye movement observations. Amygdala, recorded unilaterally in two patients and bilaterally in three, most frequently paralleled cortex in showing delta activity during stage 4 and low voltage, fast frequency activity during stage rem. Quite often, however, the delta activity might suddenly disappear unilaterally or bilaterally from amygdala in the middle of a stage 4 period or might appear during a rem period. In the one case in which uncus was recorded, uncal activity continued rhythmically in the delta frequency band throughout all stages of sleep though its activity returned to low voltage, fast frequency with awakening.

During stage rem, most limbic electrodes showed activity similar to neocortex. Some limbic sites showed sustained or intermittent rhythmic activity between 2 and 5 cps. The location of these sites varied markedly from patient to patient, but included anterior pes hippocampus and hippocampal gyrus, and anterior and dorsomedial thalamic nuclei. Despite marked interindividual variability, the activity in each site remained remarkably constant from rem period to rem period, and in those patients from whom two all-night recordings were available, from night to night. In some cases this slow activity was intermittently interspersed with periods of fast activity, while in other cases the rhythmic activity was continuous. Intermittent 3 cps activity in right anterior and middle hippocampal gyrus in an epileptic case is shown in Figure 11. Analysis of the right-middle hippocampus proved impossible in this case because of continuous epileptiform activity.

High amplitude, slow activity occupied most subcortical sites as well as cortex during stage 4. Several limbic sites, however, demonstrated low voltage, fast activity during stage 4 sleep periods. As was the case with the slow rhythmic activity during rem periods, this low voltage activity during stage 4 was restricted to the anterior two-thirds of the hippocampal complex. Figure 12 shows stage 4 from a schizophrenic patient. Both anterior hippocampal gyri demonstrate low voltage, fast activity, as does the left dorsomedial thalamic nucleus. Other thalamic nuclei show basic high voltage, slow activity but contain many brief periods of intermittent fast activity. Throughout nonrem sleep, an unusual wave consisting of a slight upward deflection, a deeply curved downward deflection, and then another upward wave, occurred in the hippocampal complex. Present in most of the epileptic cases and in both schizophrenic patients, this wave form is circled in Figure 12. The occurrence of this wave was most frequent during stage 2 when it was often bilateral and simultaneous with a cortical K-complex.

COMPARISON OF HUMAN AND CHIMPANZEE SLEEP

We will compare human and chimpanzee sleep in three separate areas: general sleep patterns, first versus last rem periods, and depth electrode recordings.

The general sleep patterns of chimpanzees are quite similar to human sleep patterns. In both species a long nonrem period usually precedes the first rem period; the first rem period is usually shorter in duration than subsequent periods; most of the stage 4 occurs early in the night; and the nonrem periods of the morning are almost pure stage 2. Rem percentage is similar in the two species. The total sleep is longer in the chimp than in man both in our own study and in the study of Bert et al. (1970). Studies of chimpanzee behavior in the wild indicate that these animals retire to arboreal sleeping nests just before sunset and arise just after sunrise (Goodall, 1962, 1963), and if labo-

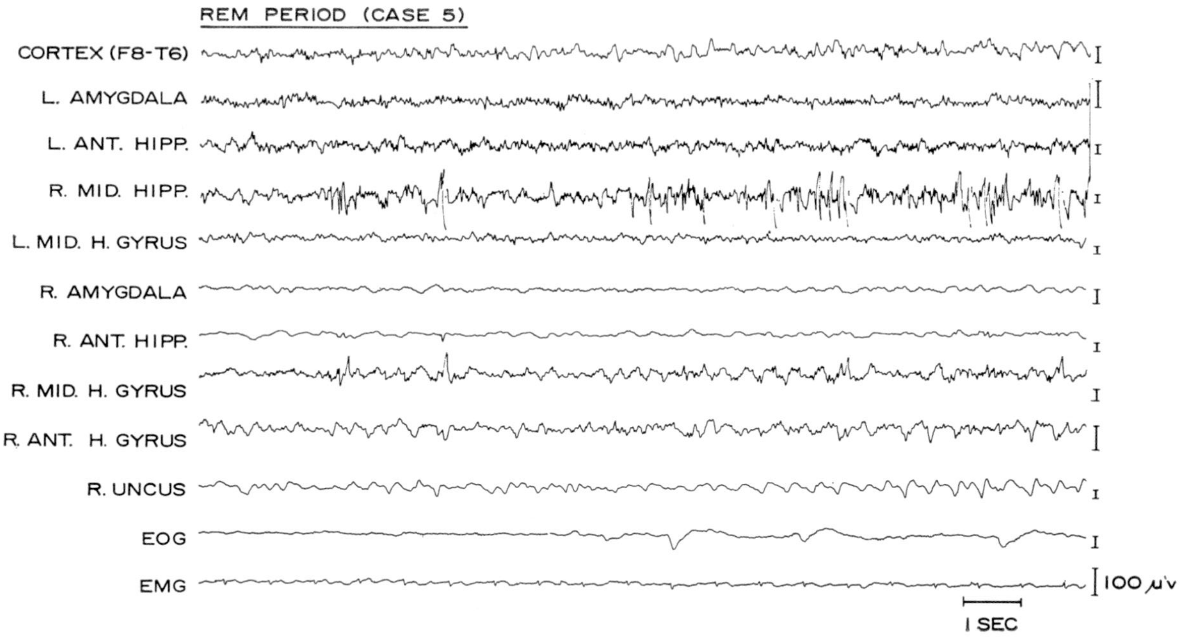

REM PERIOD (CASE 5)

CORTEX (F8-T6)
L. AMYGDALA
L. ANT. HIPP.
R. MID. HIPP.
L. MID. H. GYRUS
R. AMYGDALA
R. ANT. HIPP.
R. MID. H. GYRUS
R. ANT. H. GYRUS
R. UNCUS
EOG
EMG

100 μν

1 SEC

Figure 11. Rem sleep in an epileptic patient. Rhythmic slow activity occurs in right hippocampal gyrus (anterior and middle portions) and in uncus. From Freemon and Walter (1970).

HVS SLEEP (CASE 8)

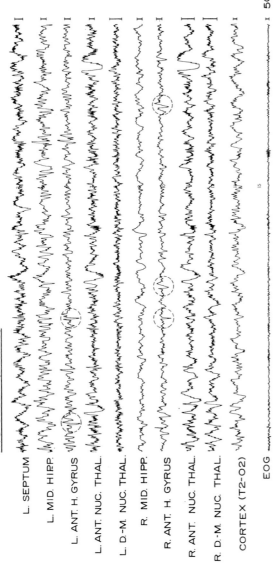

L. SEPTUM

L. MID. HIPP.

L. ANT. H. GYRUS

L. ANT. NUC. THAL.

L. D.-M. NUC. THAL.

R. MID. HIPP.

R. ANT. H. GYRUS

R. ANT. NUC. THAL.

R. D.-M. NUC. THAL.

CORTEX (T2-O2)

EOG

50μV

1 SEC

Figure 12. Nonrem stage 4 sleep in a schizophrenic patient. A characteristic waveform (circled) occurs in hippocampus. Low voltage, fast frequency activity occupies the left dorsomedial thalamic nucleus and both anterior hippocampal pyri. From Freemon and Walter (1970).

ratory chimpanzees had an earlier lights-on time and a later lights-out, the total sleep time would probably be less. In the chimpanzee, as in man, the last rem period is longer in duration and has more frequent eye and body movements than the first rem period. Table IX summarizes this comparison. The chimpanzee has saw-tooth waves morphologically indistinguishable from saw-tooth waves during human rem periods. These saw-tooth waves in chimpanzees are more frequent in later than in earlier rem periods; this is not surprising since the waveform is associated with eye movements which are also more frequent in later periods. In the chimpanzee the EMG of the posterior neck muscles does not change as the animal passes from nonrem to rem sleep, while in man the transition is associated with a marked decrease of the resting activity of the muscles of the chin. This difference may be more a function of electrode placement than a true phylogenetic difference between the sleep of the two species.

When one compares depth electrical activity from the chimpanzee with that rcorded from human patients, many similarities are apparent. In both species the amygdala shows a wide variety of types of activity which change almost independently of sleep stages which are scored on the basis of cortical activity. The computer studies of Brazier (1968) have shown an absence of coherence between cortical waveforms and activity recorded from amygdala and other limbic locations in man. We did not see any waveform in human amygdala which resembled the bursts of 21 to 24 cps activity seen in amygdala of two chimpanzees during excited wakefulness and some rem periods. However, Lesse and his co-workers (1955) noted bursts of 26 cps activity in the human amygdala during periods when the patients recalled "specific emotionally significant memories." Another similarity between these two species is the occurrence in hippocampus during nonrem sleep of a characteristic triphasic wave. This waveform is morphologically indistinguishable between the two species. Compare Figure 8 with Figure 12. In both species arousal from nonrem sleep frequently causes hippocampal desynchronization to precede cortical. This phenomenon is discussed in Chapter 6.

In man, certain brain regions contain slow waves during periods when most brain sites contain fast activity, and fast activity occupies some of these same regions during nonrem stage 4 sleep when slow activity occurs in most of the brain. This reciprocity of slow and fast activity in rem and nonrem does not occur in the chimpanzee. A number of other studies of depth electrical activity in human patients, mostly temporal lobe epileptics, have noted slowing in anterior hippocampal leads during rem sleep. Greenberg and Pearlman (1968) reported unsustained theta activity in temporal lobe epileptics. Bancaud and co-workers (1964) noted a rhythmical 7 to 8 cps activity in hippocampus during rem in a large number of temporal lobe epileptics. In a study which did not recognize sleep stages, Kajtor et al. (1957) noted that during human sleep the hippocampus frequently contained rhythmic slow activity when insular cortex had low voltage, fast frequency activity and vice versa. Markham, Walter, and Chapman (1972) studied fourteen patients with temporal lobe seizures or cerebellar tremor including the same patients whose records I examined. They noted that in both disorders 4 to 6 cps rhythmic activity occurred in amygdala, hippocampus, and nucleus ventralis lateralis of the thalamus during rem sleep. During slow wave sleep, some fast activity was described in amygdala, nucleus ventralis lateralis, and putamen. Wilson and Nashold (1969) recorded depth activity from patients suffering from intractable pain and did not note any slow activity during rem nor fast activity during slow wave sleep.

One must question whether this electrophysiologic phenomena is a difference between man and chimpanzee or a difference between normality and abnormality, between normal chimpanzee and human patients suffering temporal lobe epilepsy. Bickford (1964) suggested three methods to help elucidate normal human depth electrical activity from the study of abnormal humans: the general "normality" of the appearance of the waveforms, comparison between patients with different diseases, and comparison with depth studies in normal animals. There is nothing inherently pathological in the appearance of this reciprocal slowing; in fact, any spiking was eliminated from analysis. The phenomenon of reciprocity appears in schizophrenics as well as temporal lobe epileptics and may also occur in persons with cerebellar tremor (Markham et al., 1972) though it was not observed in persons suffering intractable pain (Wilson and Nashold, 1969). Though it does not occur in the chimpanzee, hippocampal theta during rem and fast activity in some sites during nonrem sleep is prominent in the cat, rabbit, and other species (summarized in Chapter 3).

Choice of sleeping location is another major difference between sleep of chimpanzee and of man. Chimpanzees in the wild, even though they may spend the entire day foraging on the ground, always sleep in trees (Goodall, 1962, 1963). Even the most primitive men such as the Australian aborigine or the Kalahari bushman sleep on the ground (Thomas, 1959). The final chapter of this monograph speculates on possible correlations between these two differences, one electrical and one behavioral, between the sleep of these two species. Table X summarizes some of the similarities and differences between sleep of man and sleep of chimpanzee.

In general, the similarities between human and chimpanzee sleep are very marked. Rem sleep in man must be homologous to rem sleep in the chimpanzee and is probably homologous to rem sleep in the monkey, cat, and other animals. Comparison of sleep of man and cat reveals that these two species have at least one phenomenon in common, hippocampal theta rhythm during rem, that is not seen in subhuman primates.

TABLE X

COMPARISON OF HUMAN AND CHIMPANZEE SLEEP

Similarities:

The overall sleep pattern is quite similar between the two species.

Nonrem stages 3 and 4 occur early in the night.

Later rem periods are longer and have more eye and body movements.

About 20 percent of the sleeping time is spent in the rem state.

Adaption to the laboratory distorts the sleep pattern on the first laboratory night.

The immature has a greater sleep time and higher rem time than the adult.

The cortical or scalp EEG during nonrem sleep permits division of this sleep state into four substages.

The cortical or scalp EEG during rem sleep shows theta activity and sawtooth waves.

These sawtooth waves frequently precede an eye movement.

A characteristic triphasic wave occurs in hippocampal complex during nonrem sleep.

Hippocampal desynchronization frequently precedes cortical during arousal from nonrem sleep.

Differences:

The EMG does not differentiate between nonrem and rem sleep in chimpanzee (probably related to electrode placement)

Total sleep time is longer in chimpanzee (probably related to lighting schedule).

Sharp, high voltage waveforms occur in chimpanzee hippocampus during wakefulness and nonrem sleep (unexplained).

Some subcortical sites in man but not chimpanzee show slow activity during rem sleep and fast during nonrem.

In the wild, chimpanzees always sleep in trees (an explanation relating these last two species differences is offered in the final chapter).

Chapter 5

SLEEP DEPRIVATION

His condition during the hearing alternated between apathy and an unnatural, glassy wakefulness. Only once did he actually become unconscious; he often felt on the brink of it, but a feeling of pride always saved him at the last minute. He would light a cigarette, blink, and the hearing would go on. At times he was surprised that he was able to stand it. But he knew that lay opinion set far too narrow limits to men's capacity of physical resistance; that it had no idea of their astonishing elasticity. He had heard of cases of prisoners who had been kept from sleeping for 15 to 20 days, and who had stood it.

KOESTLER, *Darkness at Noon*

TOTAL SLEEP DEPRIVATION

EVERYONE is familiar from personal experience with the subjective sensations of mild sleep loss: feeling of fatigue, heaviness of eyelids, burning of the eyes, headache or the sensation of a tight hatband. Neurological examination of individuals awake for sixty hours shows weakness of neck flexion, hand tremor, awkwardness, nystagmus, ptosis, dysarthria, poverty of facial movement, short attention span, and an apathetic appearance (Sassin, 1970). These individuals cannot read or even watch television because of visual discomfort and difficulty in concentrating. After several days without sleep, the volunteer may imagine halos around objects or cobwebs on the floor. This visual distortion sometimes progresses to frank visual hallucinations. In some individuals, paranoid ideation becomes prominent. Neurological examination at this time discloses slurring of speech, loss of ocular convergence, inability to concentrate, episodes of disorientation to time, and immediate memory loss, such as forgetting the task at hand (Ross, 1965; Kollar et al., 1968). The description of psychological changes during sleep deprivation is frustrated by a number of additional variables including the volunteer's premorbid personality, the atmosphere of the experimental situation

72

(the more supportive the milieu, the less paranoid the patient), the individual's motivation, his age, and other environmental factors. Time variables other than duration of wakefulness confound evaluation: the volunteer functions more poorly at night, when some of his circadian rhythms continue as if he were asleep, than during the day; feelings of drowsiness come in waves lasting one to three hours with superior performance between these periods of increased fatigue; and the patient frequently suffers momentary lapses of contact with environment. Formal testing is made difficult by the sleep-deprived volunteer's ability to increase his mental abilities temporarily during a period of personality or performance testing. The most boring and the longest test situations are the poorest performed by sleep-deprived individuals. Though the exact symptoms produced by sleep deprivation depend on additional variables, the sleep-deprived person is not normal, suffering both neurological and psychological deterioration (Bliss et al., 1959; Morris et al., 1960; Gulevich et al., 1966; Lubin, 1967; Wilkinson, 1968).

A number of laboratory abnormalities occur during prolonged wakefulness. The scalp electroencephalogram shows a slight decrease in the background alpha rhythm, a nonspecific EEG change seen in many conditions from Zen trance (Kasamatsu and Hirai, 1966) to alcoholic intoxication (Freemon et al., 1971). The rise in serum creatinine phosphokinase during sleep deprivation may be due to continued activity of skeletal muscles without the restorative effect of sleep and physical inactivity (Kupfer et al., 1970a). Other metabolic changes during prolonged wakefulness include a marked fall in plasma iron levels (Kuhn et al., 1967) and a moderate decline in plasma cholesterol with slight increases in circulating levels of glucose and cortisol (Kollar et al., 1969).

Deprivation of sleep contributes to the mental changes seen in the combat soldier. Descriptions of exhausted soldiers forced to stay awake in order to stay alive occur throughout literature. S.L.A. Marshall (1962) interviewed the survivors of the parachute jump into Normandy in 1944 and reported some of the symptoms of sleep deprivation in these men:

> They were dull-eyed, bodily worn and too tired to think connectedly. Even a 30 minute flop on the turf with the stars for a blanket would have doubled the power of this body and quickened the minds of its

leaders to ideas on which they had blanked out. But no one thought to take that precaution. The United States Army is indifferent toward common-sense rules by which the energy of men may be conserved in combat. These men had too little time to find their positions and check their weapons. Said Captain Patch of his people on the far right, "They were so beat that they could not understand words even if an order was clearly expressed. I was too tired to talk straight. Nothing I heard made a firm impression on me. I spoke jerkily in phrases because I could not remember the thoughts which had preceded what I said." (Marshall, *Night Drop*, 1962, p. 323)

Since World War II the U.S. Army has supported research to find chemicals which can increase the efficiency of sleep-deprived soldiers. Amphetamines can temporarily improve the performance of fatigued individuals on rote tasks (Weiss and Laties, 1962) while scopolamine and LSD typically increase the mental disorganization of sleep deprivation (Safer, 1970a, b). Of course, the best treatment for sleep deprivation is sleep. In the Vietnam War the U.S. Army has usually been able to airlift troops out of combat areas before the appearance of sleep deprivation symptoms. This may be one of the reasons for the low rate of psychiatric casualties in this conflict.

Sleep deprivation symptoms also occur in interns and other house-staff physicians. Dr. X recorded in his book *The Intern* how chronic sleep loss made him feel "constantly, chronically, unremittingly tired." Some of the bonehead errors he relates might have been due to the mental lapses of sleep deprivation. In a formal study of sleep deprivation in house staff physicians, Friedman et al. (1971) found that sleep-deprived interns misdiagnosed arrhythmias on electrocardiographic recordings more frequently than the same interns when rested.

Forced sleep deprivation has been used throughout history to break down prisoners. From the Roman execution of Perseus by the *tortura insomniae* to the all-night interrogation of Edgar Smith (1968) by the New Jersey police, the sleep-deprived have been more willing to confess than the rested. Credit for the most complete development of sleep deprivation as an applied science probably goes to Nikolai Yezhov, who was entrusted by Stalin with the interrogation of the old guard Soviet communists tried for treason in the late 1930s. Though complete details remain unpublished, it is thought that Yezhov developed the technique of sleep deprivation for ninety straight hours followed by interrogations after very brief periods of sleep. The minds of the suspects became so deranged by this prolonged treatment that they not only confessed to absurd charges like sabotaging the Soviet state by putting tacks in butter, but they came to believe that they had actually committed the offenses to which they confessed. Those readers who believe in poetic justice may appreciate that Yezhov later offended Stalin and, like Guillotine, he perished by the very technique that he had himself invented.

Recovery from total sleep deprivation is associated with increased total sleep time, a marked increase in the percentage of sleep spent in nonrem stages 3 and 4, and a marked increase in arousal threshold during all sleep stages (Berger and Oswald, 1962a; Williams et al., 1964). While total rem time is increased on the first recovery night, rem percentage is unchanged or only slightly elevated (Kales et al., 1970g). On subsequent recovery nights rem percentage is significantly increased. These increases in nonrem stage 4 and in rem sleep are accompanied by a decrease in the amount of nonrem stage 2.

REM SLEEP DEPRIVATION

If a sleeper is awakened every time he enters the rem state, he begins to enter rem sleep more frequently and must be awakened more often and more vigorously. When subsequently allowed to sleep undisturbed, he obtains more rem sleep than he did on baseline nights prior to the rem deprivation procedure. Several technical difficulties complicate the interpretation of this rem rebound. Since the early morning hours contain a greater percentage of rem sleep than the hours just after retiring, individuals who sleep longer, all other things being equal, will have a higher rem percentage than shorter sleepers (Verdone, 1968). A portion of the rem rebound, therefore, could be due to the fact that the total sleep time is longer on recovery than on baseline nights. Some studies have used pharmacological techniques to augment the rem deprivation of rem awakenings (Vogel and Traub, 1968). The rebound recorded in these studies could be due to the withdrawal of the rem suppressant drugs (see Chapter 7). Different workers have used different control nights, some using baseline nights prior to any experimental manipulation while others used recovery nights following nonrem awakenings, equal in number to rem awakenings, allowing a control for the nonspecific effect of sleep interruption. As summarized in Table XI, however, most studies have recorded

TABLE XI

REM REBOUND AFTER REM DEPRIVATION

Type of Subject	Control Rem Percentage %	Deprivation Nights (n)	Recovery Rem Percentage %	Reference
Normal	20	5	27	Dement (1960)
Normal	22	6	33	Kales et al. (1964)
Normal	20	10	38	Kales et al. (1964)
Normal	22	3	28	Sampson (1965)
Normal	24	3	26	Cartwright et al. (1967)
Schizophrenic	23	7	36	Vogel & Traub (1968)
Depressed	14	10	19	Vogel et al. (1968)
Normal	21	1	23	Foulkes et al. (1968)

a substantially increased rem percentage during recovery from rem sleep deprivation.

On the basis of this type of data, a "need" for rem sleep has been postulated. Dement, Greenberg, and Klein (1966) presented evidence that a deficit of rem sleep can be carried for several days. Volunteers were rem deprived for five nights, then allowed rem sleep only equal to baseline rem values for the next five nights. When then allowed to sleep undisturbed, these volunteers showed an increased rem percentage, suggesting that a rem deficit, like a financial debt, can be carried forward over a significant time interval. Other workers have suggested that the multiple interruptions of the rem state, rather than the actual decreased amount of time spent in rem sleep, is responsible for the rem rebound (Sampson, 1965).

The early rem deprivation studies suggested that psychological changes could occur in rem-deprived individuals, changes such as irritability (Dement, 1960), ravenous appetites (Dement and Fisher, 1963), and increased oral behavior and oral symbolism in thinking (Fisher, 1965). Kales and his co-workers (1964) found no psychological changes in long-term rem deprivation. No worsening of the clinical state occurs during rem deprivation in schizophrenic (Vogel and Traub, 1968) or depressed patients (Vogel et al., 1968). Total abolition of rem sleep for weeks by the monoamine oxidase inhibitor phenelzine does not cause any psychological abnormalities (Wyatt et al., 1971b). In a review of the literature, Vogel (1968) concluded that rem deprivation produces no psychological deficits in waking life and suggested that the earlier findings had been due to the subconscious communication to the experimental subjects of the expectations of the experimenters. Vogel emphasized that formal psychological testing had uncovered no consistent abnormalities in rem-deprived volunteers. Individuals suffering the unquestionable psychological changes due to total sleep deprivation can frequently muster their faculties to perform adequately on formal tests; one might suspect the same phenomenon could occur during rem deprivation. Sampson (1966) found that three nights of rem deprivation did not change the scores of six subjects on formal psychological tests such as the MMPI. Nevertheless, his volunteers reported changes in their behavior. All six had increased appetites. One had the sudden desire for roast duck, so he impulsively bought a duck and roasted it. Changes occurred over the course of the three nights of rem deprivation in the mental content of the brief periods of rem sleep obtained prior to each awakening; the rem mentation became more bizarre and was more frequently associated with aggression. Clemes and Dement (1967) reported that rem-deprived subjects showed changes on projective tests such as ink-blot tests and the type of test where the subject makes up a story after looking at a picture. Their conclusion that rem deprivation caused "an elevation in intensity of need and feeling and a depression of certain ego controls" means little to non-psychologists. Agnew and co-workers (1967) reported that rem deprivation caused subjects to become suspicious, withdrawn, and introspective. These same individuals, when deprived of nonrem stage 4 by shock stimulation whenever more than five delta waves appeared in one minute of the ongoing EEG, also became withdrawn but showed hypochondriasis and decreased aggression. Greenberg and his co-workers (1970) confirmed the fact that rem deprivation causes no deficit on cognitive psychological tests but may produce changes in projective tests. Their rem-deprived volunteers showed poor reality testing, greater orality, and suggestions of homosexuality during inkblot and other projective tests.

Empson and Clarke (1970) have implicated rem sleep in memory consolidation in man. They studied twenty students in pairs. At 2100 in the sleep laboratory two experimental subjects listened to a tape recording of nonsense phrases. After they had retired, one student was chosen to be rem deprived. Whenever he entered a rem period, both subjects were awakened. The rem-deprived subjects showed less recall of the tape-recorded material the next morning than did their cohorts awakened the same number of times but from random sleep stages.

A method of rem depriving experimental animals has been devised which takes advantage of the marked relaxation of the posterior neck muscles during the rem state. If an animal is placed on a small pedestal surrounded by water, he can obtain nonrem sleep; however, when he enters rem sleep his head droops, his snout splashes into the water, and he may slip off the pedestal. Using either this method of rem deprivation or the classic method of arousing an animal when his polygraphic record indicates he is entering the rem state, a rem rebound during recovery has been shown in the monkey (Berger and Meier, 1966), cat (reviewed by Dement et al., 1967), rabbit (Khazan and Sawyer, 1963), and rat (Morden et al., 1967). Rem-deprived experimental animals show clear and reproducible behavioral effects including increased motor activity and exploratory behavior (Boyaner, 1970; Albert et al., 1970) and hypersexuality as shown by the deprived animals mounting male animals or animals of other species (Dement, 1969). Rem deprivation may interfere with the retention of a conditioned avoidance response (Fishbein, 1970, 1971; Leconte and Bloch, 1970). The seizure threshold to electroconvulsive shock decreases following rem deprivation in the rat (Owen and Bliss, 1970), mouse (Cohen and Dement, 1970), and cat (Cohen et al., 1967, 1970). All these symptoms of rem deprivation disappear after the animal is allowed to sleep undisturbed.

In summary, man and experimental animals can be deprived of the complete rem state. During recovery from this deprivation procedure, an increased amount of rem sleep is obtained. In experimental animals, but not man, clear and reproducible symptoms occur during waking which are probably due to the loss of the rem state and which disappear following rem recovery. Many workers have concluded that rem deprivation causes no psychological changes whatsoever in man. It is my opinion that this conclusion is premature. Rem deprivation, like total sleep deprivation, may cause intermittent psychological dysfunction which is not picked up by formal psychological testing. Different people with different personality types may react differently to rem deprivation. Rem deprivation may not only change the deprived subject's waking behavior, it may also change his nonrem sleep. Dement (1969) has suggested that the psychological symptoms which appear in rem-deprived cats are not due to deprivation of the complete rem state but only to certain phasic components of rem sleep such as the PGO waves. Rem deprivation in man may produce dispersal of these poorly understood phasic phenomena into waking and into nonrem sleep. The psychologic response to rem deprivation in man forms one of the most challenging areas of sleep research.

BIOCHEMICAL CHANGES DURING SLEEP

Two separate neurochemical problems confront sleep research:

1. To determine the neurotransmitter substances involved in the neural structures which initiate and control sleep.

2. To discover brain metabolites synthesized during sleep for use in waking or degraded during sleep after accumulation during waking. The approach to the first problem involves the measurement of sleep stage changes after the administration of agents which effect the synthesis or degradation of neurotransmitters in the central nervous system. These studies have been discussed in Chapter 3. Studies attacking the second problem measure the level of brain metabolites during sleep or following rem deprivation or total sleep deprivation.

The biochemist conceives that sleep's function is to replenish unknown metabolites depleted during wakefulness (or degrade toxins synthesized as a side product during waking) and he conceives his mission to be the discovery and characterization of these unknown metabolites. One neurochemical substance synthesized at greater rate during sleep than during waking may be the neurotransmitter acetylcholine. Telencephalic acetylcholine falls during rem deprivation but rises during total sleep deprivation (Bowers et al., 1966; Tsuchiya et al., 1969). No change occurs in levels of acetylcholine in diencephalon or brain stem during rem deprivation or total sleep deprivation. Richter and Crossland (1949) found that a cholinergic substance, measured by acetylcholine bio-assay, was higher in whole brain extract of cats who had slept for about thirty minutes than in waking cats. Acetylcholine leaks from the neocortex during wakefulness at a much greater rate than during nonrem sleep; during rem sleep, however, the cortical release of acetylcholine rises to waking levels (Jasper and Tessier, 1971).

Other neurotransmitters may be synthesized more rapidly during sleep than during waking. The diencephalic concentration of serotonin or 5-hydroxytryptamine decreases following total sleep deprivation but not following rem deprivation (Tsuchiya et al., 1969). If an animal is allowed to sleep for only thirty minutes after twenty-four hours of sleep deprivation, his diencephalic content of serotonin is not only replenished but actually rises above control values. Intracisternal injection of labelled tryptophan during rem deprivation produces greater incorporation of radio-active label into brain serotonin than injection in control animals (Hery et al., 1970). Weiss et al. (1968) have presented preliminary evidence that the rate of serotonin turnover is increased during rem deprivation. A decreased turnover of norepinephrine occurs during rem deprivation (Pujol et al., 1968), but this same biochemical phenomenon occurs in other types of stress (Mark et al., 1969). An increase in the total brain content of a number of animo acids including aspartic acid, glutamic acid, glutamine, phenylalanine, tyrosine, valine, leucine, and isoleucine follows rem deprivation by the pedestal method (Davis et al., 1969). Regional differences occur in the biochemical response to rem deprivation. Aspartic acid content rises in frontal cortex, thalamus, reticular formation, and caudate nucleus but is unchanged in occipital cortex or superior and inferior colliculi; the inhibitory neurotransmitter gamma-aminobutyric acid rises in frontal cortex, thalamus, and reticular formation but falls in caudate nucleus and colliculi following rem deprivation (Micic et al., 1967).

The brain has a high rate of protein synthesis. Protein and peptide synthesis is higher in the sleeping than in the waking brain. When radioactively labelled leucine is injected intraperitoneally into rats which have been totally sleep deprived for eighteen hours, incorporation of label into brain protein is considerably higher in animals allowed to sleep for two hours than in animals sleep deprived for two additional hours (Rodden et al., 1970). Reich and his co-workers (1967) injected labelled phosphate into newborn rats and measured radioactivity in several brain metabolites which contain phosphate groups. They found that brain phosphoproteins from animals allowed to sleep have a higher incorporation of radioactive label than the same fraction from animals kept awake between injection and sacrifice. This is not true for liver phosphoproteins, nor is any difference apparent in the incorporation of phosphate into phospholipids or nucleic acids in brain or liver between sleeping and waking animals. Rakic and co-workers (1966) also reported increased phosphate incorporation into polypeptides in the brain of sleeping animals. In adult animals, Vitale-Neugebauer and her co-workers (1970) found a different sedimentation pattern for RNA from waking animals than from animals in nonrem sleep. Enzyme proteins have also been suggested as this hypothetical entity which is replenished by sleep. Hyden and Lange (1965) reported that the activity of the enzyme succinoxidase is high in neurons and low in glia of the brain stem during sleep, but the reverse is true during wakefulness.

Another suggestion is that energy compounds are utilized during wakefulness and replenished during sleep. Whole brain ATP, creatine phosphate, and glucose are higher in sleeping than in sleep-deprived animals (Van den Noort and Brine, 1970). Brain lactate levels are lower during sleep than during wakefulness (Cook, 1967). Karadzic and Mrsulja (1969) analyzed the brain content of glycogen following seventy-two hours of rem sleep deprivation. Rem deprivation decreases the glycogen content of caudate nucleus, hippocampal complex, and caudal brain stem but not neocortex. During three hours of recovery sleep, however, glycogen falls in neocortex and decreases further in the other brain regions but returns to normal levels after six hours of recuperative sleep. Mrsulja and Rakic (1970) reported that rem deprivation decreases glycogen content of caudate nucleus, thalamus, and hypothalamus but that atropine, propanolol, or reserpine given prior to rem deprivation blocks this glycogen-depleting effect.

From these results, it appears that many biochemical changes occur in the brain during both types of sleep. The hypothetical substance depleted by wakefulness and replenished by sleep is most likely several substances. Whatever biochemical processes occur in neurons during sleep, we know they are energy requiring. In normal sleep, unlike coma, cerebral blood flow and oxygen consumption do not fall. Using a heat clearance method, Baust (1967) found a decreased blood flow to midbrain and an increased blood flow to pontine and medullary reticular formation during rem sleep. An increase in blood flow to most brain regions during rem and a slight decrease during nonrem has been recorded with an autoradiographic technique by Reivich et al. (1968). In man, oxygen consumption and cerebral blood flow do not change during the passage from relaxed wakefulness to nonrem sleep (Mangold et al., 1955). Brebbia and Altschuler (1965) found total body oxygen consumption to be highest during rem sleep and lowest during nonrem stages 3 and 4. The first suggestion that blood flow might be increased during a specific type of sleep probably belongs to Hammond (1883, p. 145) who reported "the case of a man who, some time after receiving a severe injury of the head by which a considerable portion of the skull was lost, came under my professional care. Standing by his bedside one evening just after he had gone to sleep, I observed the scalp rise slightly from the chasm in which it was deeply depressed. I was sure he was going to awake, but he did not, and very soon he became restless and agitated while continuing to sleep. Presently he began to talk, and it was evident that he was dreaming. In a few minutes the scalp sank down to its ordinary level when he was asleep, and he became quiet. I called his wife's attention to the circumstance and desired her to observe this condition thereafter when he slept. She subsequently informed me that she could always tell when he was dreaming from the appearance of the scalp."

Chapter 6

AROUSAL

If infantry and cavalry happened to bivouac together, dawn would reveal an oddity. Cavalry was always awakened by bugle calls, but the morning summons to infantry was the long roll beaten on the drums. The cavalrymen would sleep soundly through the beating of the drums but would rouse instantly when their own bugles sounded, while it was just the other way around with infantry; bugles would not awaken them, but they got up at once when the drums began to beat. Sometimes a wakeful battery would fire a few salvos in the night, and get answering salvos from an unseen Rebel battery, and the troops would remain asleep. But the same men would come out of their blankets at once, fumble for their muskets, and fall into line if a few musket shots were fired by their own pickets.

BRUCE CATTON, *A Stillness at Appomattox*

ASCENDING RETICULAR ACTIVATING SYSTEM

THE anatomical extent of the brain stem reticular formation (RF) is defined by the lacy, reticular appearance of intertwined neuronal processes in the central portions of the medulla, midbrain, and pontine tegmentum. Circumscribed cellular groupings such as the red nucleus and cranial nerve nuclei are excluded from RF; some diffuse neuronal aggregates with separate names such as the nucleus reticularis pontis oralis or caudalis or the raphe nuclei are usually included within the anatomically defined RF (Brodal, 1969). RF neurons have a disc-oriented diffuse dendritic projection. The axon of each neuron bifurcates, descending to lower medulla and spinal cord and ascending to terminate in periacqueductal gray, subthalamus, hypothalamus, and nonspecific thalamic nuclei (Scheibel and Scheibel, 1958).

Electrical stimulation of the pontine and midbrain RF during nonrem sleep causes fast activity to replace slow waves in neocortical EEG, and the animal wakens (Moruzzi and Magoun, 1949). Lesions destroying midbrain RF destroy the electrographic and awakening effects of pontine stimulation and of peripheral pain stimulation; lesions which cut the classical sensory pathways such as the spinothalamic tract, but which spare RF, do not interfere with this arousal response (Lindsley et al., 1950; French et al., 1952). These experimental findings led to the concept of the ascending reticular activating system. This concept proposed the existence of a multisynaptic relation of neurons of the brain stem RF with the neurons of nonspecific thalamic nuclei: the nucleus centrum medianum, the interlaminar and reticular nuclei, and certain other thalamic nuclei which were thought to project diffusely to the neocortex. Increased excitation in the brain stem RF led, it was suggested, to increased excitation of neurons of the nonspecific thalamus, which led in turn to excitation of cortical neurons and wakefulness. Since sleep is known to be facilitated by a decrease in environmental stimuli, a quiet and dark room for example, sleep was thought to result from a dampening of the input to the brain stem RF, causing a decrease in activity of nonspecific thalamus and subsequently of cerebral neocortex (Magoun, 1954, 1963).

The concept of the ascending reticular activating system has been criticized. While withdrawal of peripheral sensory input may contribute to sleep induction, it cannot be the sole element in the development of sleep since many active neural and neurochemical sleep-producing mechanisms have been described (see Chapter 3). Stimulation of brain stem regions near the RF can transform ongoing cortical fast activity to slow waves, the exact opposite of the change produced by RF stimulation (Magnes, Moruzzi, and Pompeiano, 1961). The nonspecific thalamic nuclei do not project diffusely to neocortex, as postulated by the reticular activating theory in its original form; rather these nuclei project to limbic areas, to orbitofrontal cortex, and back to the brain stem RF (Scheibel and Scheibel, 1967). They may affect neocortex through interaction with specific thalamic nuclei. Many investigators noted quite early that environmental stimulation during nonrem sleep usually produces flattening of slow activity in hippocampus prior to flattening in neocortex (see the discussion following Magoun, 1954). Sometimes a minor environmental stimulus causes fast activity to appear in hippocampus transiently with little or no change in ongoing cortical slow activity (Figure 13). Environmental stimuli which awaken from nonrem sleep cause desynchronization to appear in hippocampus several seconds before fast activity replaces

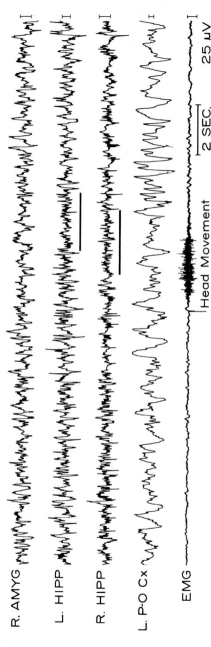

Figure 13. A chimpanzee in nonrem sleep. A brief head movement produces an electrical arousal response (replacement of slow waves by fast activity) in hippocampal leads with little change in cortical activity. From Freemon, McNew, and Adey (1969).

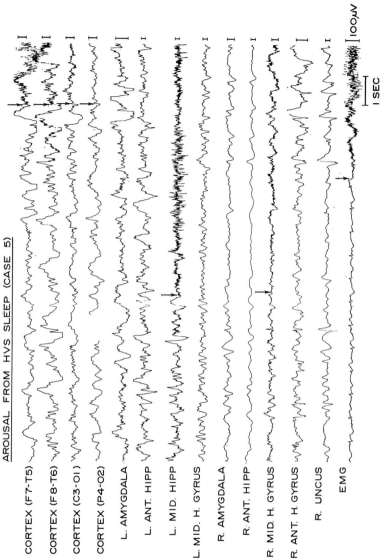

Figure 14. An epileptic patient awakens from nonrem sleep. Flattening of hippocampal activity precedes the first muscular movements which precede flattening of cortical activity. From Freemon and Walter (1970).

slow waves in neocortex (Figure 14). This phenomenon of hippocampal "arousal" preceding neocortical occurs in many species including the cat (Jouvet, 1967), chimpanzee (Freemon et al., 1969), and man (Freemon and Walter, 1970).

Brodal (1969) has presented the most devastating criticism of the concept of the ascending reticular activating system. A portion of his critique was directed at nomenclature. The word reticular refers to an anatomic region, while activating is a physiologic term. He objected to the juxtaposition of these words since the full extent of the RF was not known to participate in the activating response while arousal mechanisms certainly involved portions of the brain outside the anatomically delineated reticular structures. He also noted that portions of this system projected in a caudal direction and he doubted the advisability of the use of the word ascending. He concluded by doubting that this activating system was really a neural system in the sense of the visual system or the gamma efferent system. In his meticulous destruction of the concept of "the ascending reticular activating system," the only word to which he did not object was the word "the." The present author objects to the word "the." Chapter 10 proposes the existence of two arousal systems, both of which involve portions of RF.

The concept of the ascending reticular activating system has stimulated the development of neurophysiologic sleep research, but like most theoretical constructs, from the irreducible atom to the double helix, it has proven to be an oversimplification.

CONTROL OF SENSORY INPUT

Changes in sensory pathways during sleep are deduced from the differences of the electrical activity of one portion of a sensory system evoked by stimulation of another portion of the same system. For example, the amplitude of the response evoked from lateral geniculate body by light flashes or by electrical stimulation of the optic nerve is higher during rem than during nonrem sleep. Many workers, therefore, conclude that "transmission" of visual signals through this nucleus is greater in the rem than in the nonrem state. This increased "transmission" does not necessarily mean that more information is processed by the visual system during rem. Less activity in postsynaptic neurons could indicate more selective filtering of presynaptic impulses.

The central nervous system controls auditory input in two ways. The olivocochlear bundle, an efferent pathway in predominantly afferent cranial nerve eight, can vary the sensitivity of the hair cells of the organ of Corti (Whitfield, 1968). This mechanism shows no changes between waking and sleep nor between the two stages of sleep (Irvine et al., 1970). The second method involves the contraction of the middle ear muscles, predominantly the stapedius, dampening the movement of the round window. Cranial nerve seven supplies the stapedius muscle, and it is not unusual for some patients with Bell's palsy to complain that sounds are too loud or too harsh in the ear of the affected side. The stapedius muscle is active during sleep, particularly during the eye movements of rem sleep (Baust et al., 1964). With middle ear intact, click-evoked responses in the cochlear nucleus, the first way station of auditory impulses entering the brain, are decreased in rem as compared to nonrem sleep with a further phasic decrease of response during the eye movements of the rem state (Chin et al., 1965; Dunlop and Waks, 1968). However, if the middle ear muscles are cut, the cochlear nucleus click-evoked response shows no differences between the two stages of sleep (Baust et al., 1964). Loud clicks during wakefulness and rem sleep, but not nonrem sleep, cause an electromyographic response in middle ear muscles and ablation of the auditory cortex abolishes this response (Baust and Berlucchi, 1964). It thus appears that peripheral control of auditory input occurs during rem but not nonrem sleep. Animals with this peripheral effect abolished by tenotomy of the middle ear muscles show greater amplitude click-evoked response in inferior colliculus and in cerebellum during nonrem than during rem sleep with the waking response intermediate. This is interpreted as greater "transmission" in the old or inferior colliculus part of the auditory system during the nonrem state (Berlucchi et al., 1967). The click-evoked response in the medial geniculate nucleus shows no sleep-related changes in tenotomized animals.

Synapses of the somatosensory system occur in the nuclei cuneatus and gracilis of the medulla and the ventral posterolateral (VPL) nucleus of the thalamus. Pain sensation transmitted in the spinothalamic tract bypasses the nuclei cuneatus and gracilis. Sensation from the face proceeds to the somatosensory cortex by a parallel system involving the sensory nucleus of cranial nerve five and the ventral posteromedial

(VPM) thalamic nucleus. The electrical response recorded from the nucleus cuneatus evoked by skin or peripheral nerve electrical stimulation shows no difference in amplitude between the rem and nonrem states (Carli et al., 1966), but a marked phasic decrease of "synaptic transmission" through this nucleus occurs during the eye movements of the rem state (Carli et al., 1967). Stimulation of the somatosensory pathway from the nucleus cuneatus to the VPL nucleus of the thalamus produces an evoked response in the VPL which markedly decreases during nonrem sleep but rises back to the waking level during rem sleep (Allison, 1965; Favale et al., 1965). An additional phasic increase in "transmission" through the VPL occurs during the eye movements of the rem state (Daguino et al., 1967; Casati et al., 1969). Stimulation of the VPL causes an evoked cortical response which does not change between sleep states; the somatosensory cortical response evoked by stimulation of the midbrain reticular formation is much higher during nonrem sleep than during either waking or rem sleep (Allison, 1965). The "transmission" through the cuneate nucleus, therefore, shows no tonic changes between sleep states, but is greater through the VPL during rem than during nonrem sleep. Tactile-evoked potentials in the principal sensory nucleus of cranial nerve five are increased during nonrem sleep and decreased during rem sleep (Hernandez-Peon et al., 1965).

Extensive processing of visual information occurs in the retina (Granit, 1968), but possible changes in this retinal processing during sleep have not been analyzed. Electrical stimulation of the optic nerve or optic tract evokes a response in the lateral geniculate (LG) nucleus of the thalamus. The amplitude of this response in wakefulness and in rem sleep is greater than during nonrem sleep (Frommer and Galambos, 1964; Iwama et al., 1966). The amplitude of the earliest (or so-called presynaptic) portion of this response decreases phasically during the eye movements of rem sleep (Bizzi, 1966). Microelectrode recordings show greater unit activity in lateral geniculate body evoked by light stimulus in rem than in nonrem sleep (Maffei et al., 1965; Mukhametov and Rizzolatti, 1969). These studies suggest that "transmission" through the LG nucleus is greater during rem than during nonrem sleep. Little difference occurs in visual cortex between responses evoked in rem and in nonrem sleep states by stimulation of the LG body or the visual thalamocortical radiations. The response evoked in posterior hypothalamus or midbrain tegmentum by visual stimuli differs from that evoked in LG nucleus, being of greater amplitude during nonrem than during rem sleep (Bogacz and Wilson, 1969).

The cortical evoked potential has been recorded during sleep in both experimental animals and man. In general, the short latency components of the average cortical evoked response have somewhat higher amplitude during nonrem than during rem sleep, but the latency from the stimulus to the first response does not change. The longer latency portions of the cortical evoked response are greater in amplitude and in latency during nonrem than during rem sleep (H.L. Williams et al., 1962; Nakagawa, 1965; Weitzman and Kremen, 1965; Allison et al., 1966; Desmedt and Manil, 1970). The interpretation of these findings is difficult. During wakefulness a large number of variables can change the amplitude and shape of the cortical evoked potential including attention (Guerrero-Figueroa and Heath, 1964), handedness (Eason et al., 1967), and time of day (Heninger et al., 1969). Species differences in evoked potential exist during waking (Goldring et al., 1970) and possibly during sleep (Goff et al., 1966).

In summary, the animal studies reviewed in this section demonstrate that the central nervous system controls its sensory input differently in different states of consciousness. During rem sleep the "transmission" of sense specific stimuli increases in VPL and LG nuclei of the thalamus. Peripheral control of auditory input through contraction of inner ear muscles occurs during waking and rem sleep, but this control is lost during nonrem sleep. On the other hand, "transmission" of auditory potentials through the inferior colliculus is greater during nonrem than during rem. Sensory input to the limbic system occurs during wakefulness by poorly understood pathways (MacLean et al., 1968), but the examination of the changes in sensory processing by phylogenetically older brain areas has just begun.

ENVIRONMENTAL INTERACTION DURING HUMAN SLEEP

Awareness of environmental events is decreased but not absent during sleep. Some environmental interaction can occur during sleep, though usually this is not remembered unless the sleeper is immediately awakened.

The ancient observation that meaningful stimuli awaken more readily than neutral ones, the baby's soft cry but not the loud rattle of the passing elevated train awakens the new mother, has been scientifically validated by Oswald and his co-workers (1960) and by Wilson and Zung (1966). Oswald et al. (1960) instructed subjects to awaken whenever they heard a specific name. The occurrence of the special name against a background of many other names frequently awoke the sleepers. Wilson and Zung (1966) financially rewarded sleepers who awoke following the auditory stimuli of recorded bagpipes or a telephone ringing. These volunteers were able to rouse themselves from any stage of sleep when these sounds were played, while sleeping through the occurrence of other recorded sounds such as a doorbell ringing, a vehicle passing, animal howls, and so forth. These studies indicate that the sleeper can assume a mental set to awaken upon hearing a specific stimulus and can maintain this set throughout a night's sleep. In addition, these results suggest that environmental events can be analyzed by auditory portions of the brain during sleep.

The sleeper can also perform simple motor acts during sleep on command and with subsequent memory loss for these acts. H. L. Williams et al. (1966) instructed subjects to close a switch when a specific tone sounded. If the switch was not closed, the sleeper was awakened by loud sounds and electric shocks. All subjects learned to press the switch to avoid these arousing stimuli. Frequently, the sleeper pressed the switch, which was taped to his hand, after the sounding of the tone without any change in his EEG. Though this auditory discrimination and motor act could be performed in any stage of sleep, the sleeper in general made the response better in the rem than the nonrem state. Okuma and his colleagues (1966) instructed volunteers to press a switch the same number of times that a light flashed. This type of visual discrimination and motor act could be performed in any stage of sleep. The type of mistaken response varied between stages, however. In nonrem sleep, the subject sometimes pressed the switch one or two times less than the number of light flashes. If immediately awakened, he usually reported that he had perceived the same number of flashes as the button press, that is, one or two less than the real number. On the other hand, during rem sleep the sleeper sometimes failed to press the switch at all. If immediately awakened he usually reported that he had perceived the correct number of flashes but had not pressed the switch because he had "forgotten" to do so or some aspect of rem mentation interfered with the response. Unlike these studies where the the subjects responded during sleep according to instructions received during wakefulness, Evans and his co-workers (1966, 1969, 1970) gave suggestions during the rem state, such as "whenever I say the word leg, your left leg will feel cramped and you will move it." Subjects responded to the cue word appropriately during the same rem period, later rem periods the same night, or even during rem periods on subsequent nights. There exists some evidence that a sleeper can note his entry to a rem period, presumably by subjectively noting his typical rem mentation, and can signal this knowledge by pressing a switch without awakening (Antrobus et al., 1965; Salamy, 1970).

In summary, abundant evidence shows that the sleeping human can evaluate and respond to environmental occurrences. He can carry a set in his mind, a set such as instructions to respond to a certain stimulus or a set to awaken at a certain time (Orr et al., 1968; Tart, 1970; Zung and Wilson, 1971). The maximal ability to analyze environmental events during sleep probably belonged to Norbert Weiner, as described in an editorial (1965) in *The Journal of Nervous and Mental Disease:*

> To the awe and amusement of the rest of us, he would fall asleep from time to time, head on shoulder, snoring with gusto. Suddenly the snore would be interrupted; and he would explode out of deep sleep into full sentences which had direct and incisive relevance to the discussion that had been going on around his sleeping head. This happened so often that it could not be dismissed as a chance coincidence.

DEPTH OF SLEEP

Which stage of sleep is deepest? The student asking this seemingly simple question looks at you with ingenuous anticipation, expecting a simple answer, like rem, or nonrem. As you hesitate or begin with, "well . . .," his face takes on a quizzical look and he expects a slightly more complex answer, maybe rem during eye movements or nonrem stage 4. Actually, this question opens a door on some of the most complex areas in brain research, on the centrifugal control of brain input, on the amnestic interaction of sleeper with environment, on the processing of internal rather than external stimuli, on the changes in classical pathways during sleep.

It is difficult to define sleep depth. To some, a mindless sleep, sleeping "like a log," is deeper than sleep with mental activity. As exemplified by this Christmas carol, deep equals dreamless:

> O little town of Bethlehem, how still we see thee lie;
> Above thy deep and dreamless sleep the starlit skies go by.

This introspective definition serves science poorly; it cannot be quantified. Most scientific definitions of sleep depth have involved arousal threshold. To awaken from the deepest stage of sleep requires the greatest stimulus intensity. For example, with stimulating electrodes in brain stem reticular formation, greater voltage is required to awaken from rem than from nonrem sleep, indicating the greater "depth" of the rem state (see Table XII). This same result occurs in the rat, cat, and monkey. Environmental arousal stimuli such as sounds show different results in different species. In man, nonrem slow wave sleep requires louder sounds to awaken than does rem sleep, while rem requires louder sounds than does nonrem stage two. During recovery from sleep deprivation, the arousal thresholds are markedly elevated in both states of sleep (H.L. Williams et al., 1964). Table XII summarizes many arousal threshold studies using different species, different arousal stimuli, and different definitions of awakening. Complicating this problem further is the fact that in man and in animals, meaningful stimuli awaken more readily than neutral stimuli of the same intensity level (Siegel et al., 1965). As previously discussed in Chapter 2, meaningful stimuli can be incorporated into ongoing mental activity (Berger, 1963). An additional complication is provided by the observation that night rem periods have higher arousal thresholds than rem periods occurring during daytime naps (Corvalan, 1970).

The nomenclature of sleep stages does nothing to aid our ideas of sleep depth. Many French and Italian sleep scientists working with experimental animals actually refer directly to the rem state as deep sleep and call the nonrem state light sleep. At my elbow lies a volume of the *Archives Italiennes de Biologie;* I thumb through it to see an article entitled: "Presynaptic and Postsynaptic Changes in Specific Thalamic Nuclei During Deep Sleep" (Dagnino et al., 1969). In the context of the article one can see that the authors are examining thalamic nuclei during rem sleep. On the other hand, many British and American sleep researchers working with human subjects refer to nonrem stage 4 or nonrem stages 3 and 4 together as deep sleep.

TABLE XII

AROUSAL THRESHOLD

Study	Species	Definition of Wakefulness	Arousal Stimulus	"Deepest" Stage
Okuma et al. (1966)	man	press switch	flashing light	nonrem stage 4 (rem "deeper" than stage 2).
Korner (1968)	human newborn	startle or facial grimace	sound	nonrem
Pisano et al. (1966)	man	subject speaks	pain	no difference
H. L. Williams et al. (1964)	man	press switch	sound	nonrem stage 4 (rem "deeper" than stage 2).
Keefe et al. (1971)	man	press switch; EEG change	sound	no difference
Pollak et al. (1967)	monkey	opens eyes, body movement	pontine RF midbrain RF	rem rem
Hodes and Suzuki (1965)	cat	EEG flattening, behavior	midbrain RF vestibular n. frontal cortex	rem rem nonrem
Gassel and Pompeiano (1967)	cat	EEG flattening, head movement	peripheral n.	rem
Siegel et al. (1965)	cat	EEG flattening, behavior	sound	rem
Roldan et al. (1963)	rat	EEG flattening	midbrain RF sound	rem rem

When attempting to discuss the concept of sleep depth one must define species, methods of stimulation, sensory modalities, methods of subdividing sleep states, time of night, so many variables that the concept itself begins to lose meaning. Which stage of sleep is deepest? Certainly the question cannot be answered in a simple manner; the unqualified question may be scientifically meaningless.

Chapter 7

CLINICAL PHARMACOLOGY OF SLEEP

Not poppy nor mandragora,
Nor all the drowsy syrups of the world,
Shall ever medicine thee to that sweet sleep
Which thou owed'st yesterday.

SHAKESPEARE, *Othello*

CLINICAL PHARMACOLOGY

DOES chlorpromazine increase rem sleep (Toyoda, 1964), increase delta sleep without affecting rem sleep (Lester and Guerrero-Figueroa, 1966), decrease rem sleep (Feinberg et al., 1969c), increase rem sleep only after the first night (Lewis and Evans, 1969), increase total sleep time without changing sleep stage percentages (Kupfer et al., 1971), decrease delta sleep latency without changing sleep stage percentages (Lester et al., 1971), or have no effect at all on polygraphically monitored sleep (Sagales et al., 1969)? The incomparability of results from different laboratories has driven many clinical scientists to despair the entire field of sleep pharmacology and to ignore important clinical correlations. This chapter attempts to bring this complicated field together. Since species differences in the sleep response to drugs may exist, this review restricts itself to studies in man.

The expense and laboriousness of all-night polygraphy limits the number of subjects and the number of nights which can be monitored in any single study. Some publications report drug effects in a single volunteer. Only a few laboratories have studied two different doses of the same agent. The traditional pharmacologic construction of a dose-response curve is seldom attempted in sleep research. Different effects or different doses of chlorpromazine may explain the divergent results summarized in the previous paragraph. Low doses of chlorpromazine increase rem percentage, high doses depress rem, and intermediate

96

doses do not change sleep stage percentages (see Lewis and Evans, 1969).

Drug research using rem/nonrem measurements suffers certain pitfalls peculiar to this type of investigation. In order to avoid the first night effect discussed in Chapter 1, most studies have utilized subjects acclimated to the rigors of sleeping with electrodes applied to scalp, face, and chin. Another problem is the taking of unmonitored naps or surreptitious drugs which can influence the sleep patterns during night sleep. Most investigators have simply requested their subjects to refrain from drugs and napping while a few studies of patients have utilized nurse's observations. The widespread surreptitious use of illegal drugs which may change nocturnal sleep emphasizes that the investigator must use care in the selection of subjects (Mellinger et al., 1971). These minor problems are overshadowed by three drug research dangers which, if not considered, can make a study incomprehensible. These are the nonindependence of successive nights, the lack of control for sleep length, and the failure to examine or report a portion of the data smaller than the entire night.

The nonindependence of successive nights effect was described originally by Oswald and Thacore (1963) in addicts, confirmed experimentally by Rechtschaffen and Maron (1964) and by Oswald and Priest (1965), and codified by Oswald (1968). Many drugs which decrease rem acutely tend to lose this rem suppressant effect when given over several consecutive nights. Apparently not related solely to increased drug catabolism but at least partially due to brain homeostatic mechanisms, this decreasing effect of the drug advances to a point where sleep following chronic drug administration does not differ from sleep on baseline nights. If the drug is abruptly withdrawn at this time, a marked increase in rem percentage occurs and lasts for several days. Therefore, when two drugs with the same action on the rem state are given on successive nights, the drug given first has greater effect than the one given on the second night. For example, Brannen and Jewett (1969) studied two phenothiazines, promethazine and trifluoperazine, by administering each drug alternately on two successive nights following three baseline nights. They concluded that promethazine had no effect on rem sleep while trifluoperzine increased the percentage of sleep time spent in the rem type of sleep. It is essentially impossible to decipher how much of the effect of one drug was due to its pharmacological action and how much was due to the fact that the other drug was, in half the cases, taken the previous night.

Since the early morning hours contain a higher percentage of rem sleep than the hours just after retiring in the evening (Verdone, 1968), subjects who sleep eight hours will have a slightly higher rem percentage than subjects who sleep six hours. A drug which merely increases sleep time without really changing sleep patterns at all will masquerade as an agent which increases rem sleep. Hartmann (1966) gave reserpine to six volunteers and reported that the drug increased rem percentage. The same result was obtained by Hoffman and Domino (1969) in twenty prisoners. Since reserpine also increased total sleep time in both the studies, its effect on rem might not be a specific pharmacological action. A subsequent study by H.L. Williams et al. (1969a) did control for sleep length yet showed reserpine to increase rem percentage. The usual method to control for sleep length is to cut all records to some specific value such as seven hours or the length of the shortest record. Lewis and Evans (1969) used a regression equation calculated from eighty control records to correct for increase in total sleep time; their conclusion that low doses of chlorpromazine increase rem percentage hinges on the correctness of this approach. A drug which decreases rem percentage but also increases sleep time, a common combination, will have its effect on rem obscured if the investigator fails to equate sleep duration on drug and placebo nights.

Another occasional shortcoming of drug studies is the failure to compare portions of the record smaller than the entire night. Looking at smaller portions of the record, such as halves or thirds of the night, or preferably each rem period, strongly strengthens one's power to describe the effects of a drug. For example, Muzio and his co-workers (1966) found that LSD had no effect on overall rem percentage but markedly increased the duration of either the first or second rem period, sometimes to over an hour. A distinct and characteristic effect of LSD on rem sleep would have been missed if the investigators had only looked at the single number obtained from all night recording. Several rapid-acting drugs can decrease rem percentage in the first portion of the night while the rem percentage in the second half of the night rises, so that the overall rem percentage is unchanged. One can see that this pitfall assumes particular importance if one concludes that a drug has no effect on sleep patterns.

Of the many pharmacological studies of polygraphic sleep, in only three have drug and placebo been given in a double-blind manner, with both investigator and subject unaware which tablet contained active material. In other studies, two drugs were given double-blind, but then each was compared to nights in which placebo was given single-blind, with investigator, but not subject, aware that the medication was inert. While the double-blind method has never been shown to be necessary in rem/nonrem research, a nonpolygraphic study reported that patients with mild insomnia had a more restful sleep, as judged by their own subjective reports, after placebo that was administered double-blind than after single-blind placebo (Nicolis and Silvestri, 1967). Apparently the investigators in that study subconsciously communicated their expectations of drug effect to their subjects. Much of the early research with psychoactive compounds has been discarded onto the garbage heap of science because of failure to use double-blind methodology. Some of the contradictory results in sleep pharmacology may be explained by the unconscious bias of the investigator changing the subject's sleep patterns (see Modell, 1969).

Table XIII summarizes human sleep studies measuring drug effects on rem/nonrem polygraphic measurements reported in complete form up to the middle of 1971. Abstracts are excluded as are studies of drug withdrawal in addicts and massive drug overdose. The numbered columns indicate which studies took into account the problems discussed. Column 1 indicates with a plus those studies which either separated experimental nights by more than one nondrug night or which specifically analyzed drug adaptation and subsequent withdrawal. The nonindependence of successive nights is the single greatest problem in sleep pharmacology. Column 2 indicates with a plus those studies which either indicated in their procedural description that sleep length was equated on experimental and control nights or whose results section showed approximately the same sleep duration on drug and placebo nights. Studies which conclude that a drug raises rem percentage should control for sleep length. Column 3 indicates which studies report data in amounts less than the entire night. Studies which conclude that a drug has no effect on sleep stages should examine portions of a night's sleep. Column 4 indicates with a plus double-blind studies; longitudinal sleep studies cannot in their basic design administer double-blind medication on alternate nights. Deciding which of these studies fulfilled these criteria and which did not proved difficult, and the reader may wish to consult the original articles. Nevertheless Table XIII gives an overview of sleep pharmacology's results and problems. Many of these studies have examined sleep latency, rem latency, time awake after falling asleep, number of eye movements in each rem period, and other sleep parameters. The results section of Table XIII for sake of uniformity, restricts itself to changes in the percentage of sleep time spent in rem sleep or in the substages of nonrem.

In my opinion, two valid research strategies emerge from this myriad or different approaches to sleep pharmacology. Double-blind alternation of single nights of drug and placebo separated by several nondrug nights gives the acute effect of a drug on sleep, free of any subconscious bias of the investigator. This type of design measures only the acute effect of a drug; an agent like phenelzine which has no effect on the first night it is given but has marked effects on subsequent nights, will not have its sleep properties adequately described by this design strategy. The longitudinal study of several consecutive nights precludes double-blind design but allows the analysis of chronic drug effects and of the sleep response to drug discontinuance.

BARBITURATES

A review of the results portion of Table XIII reveals that some drugs have apparently different effects on sleep when tested in different laboratories. Some of the reasons for these discrepancies have been discussed. Some pharmacologic agents have complicated interactions with sleep states which only future research of the highest caliber will be able to unravel. Other drugs, though, have sleep effects which have been clearly described by existing studies. As examples of agents with reproducible effects on sleep, alcohol and the barbiturates will be reviewed in detail.

As a class of pharmacologic agents, the barbiturates are commonly used and commonly abused. The sleeping pills pentobarbital and secobarbital are among the twenty most frequently prescribed medications in the United States (Friend, 1969). The barbiturates serve as the most common chemical causing death by suicide (F.M. Berger,

TABLE XIII
CLINICAL PHARMACOLOGY OF SLEEP

Study	Drug	Subjects	1	2	3	4	Results
Gresham et al. (1963)	Alcohol, 1 gm/kg	7 normal	0	+	+	0	Decreased rem sleep.
Oswald et al. (1963)	Heptabarbitone, 400 mg	6 normal 6 depressed	0	0	+	0	Decreased rem sleep.
Rechtschaffen and Maron (1964)	Amphetamine, 15 mg	8 normal	+	+	0	0	Decreased rem; decreased total sleep time; rem rebound upon drug withdrawal.
Toyoda (1964)	Chlorpromazine, 50 mg	6 mixed	+	+	0	0	Increased rem sleep.
	Imipramine, 50 mg						Decreased rem sleep.
Freemon et al. (1965)	Meprobamate, 1200 mg	8 normal	+	+	+	+	Decreased rem; increased stage 2.
Green (1965)	LSD, 300 mcg	1 alcoholic	+	+	+	0	Increased rem sleep.
Oswald and Priest (1965)	Amylobarbitone, 400 mg	4 normal	+	+	+	0	Decreased rem sleep; withdrawal rem rebound.
	Nitrazepam, 15 mg						Decreased rem sleep; withdrawal rem rebound.
Baekeland (1966)	Methylphenidate, 5 mg	6 normal	+	+	+	0	Decreased rem; increased stage 2.
Evans and Oswald (1966)	Tryptophan, 5 gm	7 narcoleptic	+	+	+	0	Increased rem (not an all-night recording).

Study	Drug	Subjects	1	2	3	4	Results
Hartmann (1966)	Reserpine, 2 mg	6 normal	+	0	0	0	Increased rem sleep.
Lester and Guerrero-Figueroa (1966)	Chlorpromazine, 100 mg	8 normal	+	0	+	0	Increased delta sleep.
	Alpha-chloralose, 500 mg						Decreased rem; increased delta sleep.
	Phenobarbital, 120 mg						Increased delta sleep.
	Thiopental, 300 mg IV						Decreased rem; increased delta sleep.
Muzio et al. (1966)	LSD, 30 mcg	12 normal	+	0	+	0	Increased rem in first part of night.
Oswald et al. (1966)	Tryptophan, 5 gm	16 normal	+	+	+	0	Increased rem (2 hr. recording only).
Toyoda (1966)	Atropine, 10 mg	9 mixed	+	0	+	0	No effect on sleep stages.
Yuko et al. (1966)	Alcohol, 1 gm/kg	3 normal	+	+	+	0	Decreased rem in first half of night; rem rebound on withdrawal.
Baekeland (1967)	Pentobarbital, 100 mg	20 normal	+	+	+	+	Decreased rem sleep.
	Amphetamine, 15 mg						Decreased rem sleep.
Hartmann (1967a)	Tryptophan, 120 mg/kg	8 normal	+	0	0	0	Increased rem; increased total sleep time.
Ritvo et al. (1967)	Imipramine, 50 mg	7 enuretics	0	0	0	0	Decreased rem; increased stage 2 (first drug night discarded).

Study	Drug	Subjects	1	2	3	4	Results
Yules et al. (1967)	Alcohol 1 gm/kg	4 normal	+	+	+	0	Decreased rem; rem rebound on withdrawal
Evans and Lewis, (1968)	Amylobarbitone, 400 mg	2 normal	+	+	0	0	Decreased rem; rem rebound on withdrawal; rem rebound blocked by chlorpromazine.
Hartmann (1968b)	Pentobarbital, 100 mg	8 normal	+	+	0	0	Decreased rem sleep.
	Amitryptyline, 75 mg						Decreased rem sleep.
	Chlordiazepoxide, 100 mg						No effect on sleep stages.
Knowles et al. (1968)	Alcohol, 180 ml	1 normal	+	0	+	0	Decreased rem in first half of night; rem rebound on withdrawal.
Lester et al. (1968)	Secobarbital, 200 mg	14 normal	+	0	+	0	No effect on rem; delta sleep increased in first half of night, decreased in second half.
Oswald et al. (1968)	Diethylproprion, 50 mg	6 normal	+	+	+	0	Decreased rem; withdrawal rem rebound (2 hr. recording).
	Fenfluramine, 40 mg						No effect on sleep stages (2 hr. recordings).
Torda (1968)	LSD, variable, given during third rem period.	2 normal	0	0	+	0	Decreased latency to fourth rem period.
Brannen and Jewett (1969)	Promethazine, 50 mg	7 normal	0	+	+	0	No effect on sleep stage percentages; sleep cycle length increased.
	Trifluoperazine, 5 mg						Increased rem sleep.

Study	Drug	Subjects	1	2	3	4	Results
Brebbia et al. (1969)	Lithium, 1 gm/24 hr	6 mixed	+	+	0	0	No effect on sleep stages.
Feinberg et al. (1969c)	Phenobarbital, 200 mg	6 mixed	+	+	0	0	Decreased rem sleep.
	Chlorpromazine, 200 mg						Decreased rem sleep.
Greenberg et al. (1969)	Nitrous oxide by inhalation	7 normal	+	0	0	0	No effect on sleep stages
Haider (1969)	Amylobarbitone, 200 mg	6 normal	+	+	+	0	Decreased rem; increased stage 2.
	Nitrazepam, 10 mg						Decreased rem; increased stage 2.
Hoffman and Domino (1969)	Reserpine, 0.14 mg/kg	20 prisoners	+	0	0	0	Increased rem, prolonged effect.
Kales et al. (1969)	Glutethimide, 500 mg	5 normal	+	+	0	0	Decreased rem; withdrawal rem rebound.
	Methyprylon, 300 mg	7 normal					Decreased rem; withdrawal rem rebound.
	Chloral hydrate, 500 mg	10 normal					No effect on sleep stages.
Lewis and Evans (1969)	Chlorpromazine, 25 mg	7 normal	+	?	0	0	Increased rem after the first night.
	Chlorpromazine, 100 mg						Decreased rem sleep.
Rubin et al. (1969)	Glutethimide, 1 gm	4 normal	+	0	0	0	Decreased rem sleep.

Study	Drug	Subjects	1	2	3	4	Results
Sagales et al. (1969)	Scopolamine, 0.006 mg/kg	8 normal	0	+	0	0	Decreased rem sleep.
	Chlorpromazine, 0.4 mg/kg						No effect on sleep stages.
H. L. Williams et al. (1969a)	Reserpine, 1 mg	16 normal	+	+	+	0	Increased rem on second drug night.
	Tryptophan, 7.5 gm	11 normal					Increased delta sleep.
	Phenylalanine, 7.5 gm	11 normal					Increased delta sleep.
H. L. Williams et al. (1969b)	Alpha-chloralose, 500 mg	10 normal	+	+	0	0	Decreased rem; increased delta sleep.
R. L. Williams and Agnew (1969)	Pentobarbital, 200 mg	9 normal	0	+	0	+	Decreased rem; increased stage 2.
	Meprobamate, 800 mg						No effect on sleep stages.
	Glutethimide, 500 mg						Decreased rem sleep.
	Methaqualone, 300 mg						No effect on sleep stages.
Wyatt et al. (1969a)	Parachlorophenylalanine, 4 gm/24 hr	4 carcinoid	+	0	0	0	Decreased rem with no tolerance.
Wyatt et al. (1969b)	Isoniazid, 400 mg	1 normal	+	0	+	0	No effect on sleep stages.
	Isocarboxazid, 60 mg	1 normal					Decreased rem sleep.

Study	Drug	Subjects	1	2	3	4	Results
	Mebanazine, 15 mg	1 depressed					Decreased rem; withdrawal rem rebound.
	Phenelzine, 45 mg	1 depressed					Decreased rem.
	Pargyline, 100 mg	1 normal					Decreased rem.
Zung (1969a)	Desipramine, 75 mg/24 hr	6 depressed	+	0	0		Increased delta sleep.
Zung (1969b)	Desipramine, 75 mg/24 hr	17 normal					Decreased rem and increased delta sleep on fourth day of drug.
• • •							• • •
Akindele et al. (1970)	Nialimide, 10 mg/kg	5 normal	+	0	+	0	No effect on sleep stages.
	Phenelzine, 90 mg	4 normal					Decreased rem; increased stage 2; withdrawal rem rebound.
	Phenelzine, 90 mg	3 depressed					Decreased rem; increased delta sleep.
Bricolo et al. (1970)	Levodopa, 4 gm/24 hr	14 parkinson	+	+	0	0	No effect on sleep stages.
Davison et al. (1970)	Methaqualone, 250 mg and Diphenhydramine, 25 mg	14 normal	+	+	0	0	No effect on sleep stages.
	Quinalbarbital, 100 mg and Amylobarbital, 100 mg						Decreased rem sleep.

Study	Drug	Subjects	1	2	3	4	Results
Evans and Ogunremi (1970)	Chloral hydrate, 800 mg	4 normal	0	+	0	+	Decreased rem sleep.
	Dichloralphenazone, 1.3 gm						No effect on sleep stages.
	Methaqualone, 250 mg and Diphenhydramine 25 mg						No effect on sleep stages.
Firth et al. (1970)	Fenfluramine, 40 mg	7 normal	+	+	0	0	No effect on sleep stages.
Kales et al. (1970b)	Flurazepam, 30 mg	3 insomnic	+	0	+	0	No effect on sleep stages.
	Chloral hydrate 1 gm	4 insomnic					No effect on sleep stages.
	Glutethimide, 500 mg	4 insomnic					Decreased rem; withdrawal rem rebound.
Kales et al. (1970d)	Flurazepam, 30 mg	4 normal	+	0	+	0	No effect on sleep stages.
	Flurazepam, 60 mg	not given					Decreased rem sleep.
	Chloral hydrate, 1 gm	5 normal					No effect on sleep stages.
	Methaqualone, 300 gm	5 normal					Decreased rem; withdrawal rem rebound.
	Methaqualone, 150 mg	5 normal					No effect on sleep stages.

Study	Drug	Subjects	1	2	3	4	Results
Kales et al. (1970f)	Glutethimide, 500 mg	5 normal	+	0	+	0	Decreased rem; increased stage 2; withdrawal rem rebound.
	Methyprylon, 300 mg	7 normal					Decreased rem; withdrawal rem rebound.
	Pentobarbital, 100 mg	4 normal					Decreased delta sleep.
Kupfer et al. (1970b)	Lithium, 1.8 gm/24 hr	7 manic-depressive	+	+	0	0	Decreased rem; increased delta sleep
Lewis (1970)	Fenfluramine, 40 mg	8 normal	+	+	+	0	No effect on sleep stages
	Chlorphenteramine, 50 mg						Decreased rem sleep.
	Diethylproprion, 25 mg						Decreased rem sleep.
	Amphetamine, 7.5 mg						Decreased rem; increased stage 2.
Wyatt et al. (1970a)	Levodopa, variable dose	7 movement disorder	+	0	0	0	Decreased rem sleep.
Wyatt et al. (1970b)	Tryptophan, 7.5 gm	5 normal	+	0	0	0	Decreased rem; increased delta sleep.
		7 insomnic					No effect on sleep stages.
Baekeland and Lundwall (1971)	Methyldopa, 1.25 gm/24 hr	10 normal	+	+	+	0	Increased rem and decreased delta sleep in first 3 hours only.
Coulter et al. (1971)	Reserpine, 1 mg	10 normal	+	0	0	0	Increased rem and decreased delta sleep on day after medication taken.

Study	Drug	Subjects	1	2	3	4	Results
Dunleavy et al. (1971)	Debrisoquine, 40 to 60 mg	3 normal	+	+	+	0	Decreased rem; withdrawal rem rebound.
	Guanethidine, 40 mg	2 normal					Decreased delta sleep.
	Propanolol, 120 mg	3 normal					No effect on sleep stages.
Haider and Oswald (1971)	Amylobarbitone, 200 mg	6 normal	0	+	+	0	Decreased rem; increased stage 2.
	Nitrazepam, 10 mg						Decreased rem; increased stage 2.
Hartmann et al. (1971)	Tryptophan, 120 mg/kg	10 normal	+	0	0	0	Increased rem sleep.
A. Kales et al. (1971)	Levodopa	4 parkinson	+	+	0	0	Decreased rem sleep.
		4 normal					No effect on sleep stages.
J. Kales et al. (1971)	Methapyrilene, 50 mg and Scopolamine, 0.5 mg	5 insomnic	+	0	+	0	Decreased rem in first part of night only.
Kupfer et al. (1971)	Chlorpromazine, 100 mg	9 mixed	+	0	0	0	No effect on sleep stages; increased total sleep time.
Lester et al. (1971)	Chlorpromazine, 150 mg	12 normal	+	+	0	0	No effect on sleep stages: decreased latency to first rem period.
Wyatt et al. (1971b)	Phenelzine, 60 mg/24 hr	6 mixed	+	0	0	0	Total rem suppression without tolerance.
Wyatt et al. (1971c)	5-Hydroxytryptophan, 600 mg	8 normal	+	+	0	0	Increased rem sleep.

The columns numbered 1 through 4 refer to control (+) of lack of control (0) for some major problems in drug research discussed in the text. Respectively these are nonindependence of successive nights, control for sleep length, analysis of a portion of the data less than the entire night, and double-blind administration of drug and placebo.

1967). This class of drugs has a characteristic effect on sleep.

Oswald and his co-workers (1963) were the first to study the effect of barbiturates on rem sleep in six depressed patients and six age-matched controls. In the depressives rem percentage decreased from a mean of 20.6 percent on placebo nights to 14.8 percent when amylobarbitone was given; controls showed a drop from 23.3 percent to 11.8 percent. The increase in nonrem sleep did not appear in any one of the nonrem stages but was distributed in all four. Ten of the twelve subjects took amylobarbitone in a dose of 400 mg orally while the other two, one depressive and one control, took a dose of 200 mg because the higher dose caused a subjective hangover effect. A partial alternation procedure was used, but in many cases the active agent was given two nights in a row, and all patients received amylobarbitone on the first night in the laboratory. Lester and Guerrero-Figueroa (1966) studied two barbiturates, phenobarbital and thiopental, as well as other drugs. Phenobarbital in a dose of 120 mg orally was given to four subjects and in a dose of 240 mg to two subjects. The dose of thiopental to four subjects was 300 mg intravenously. All drugs and a placebo night recorded in the laboratory were separated by a week of sleeping at home to eliminate the nonindependence of successive nights effect. Thiopental, but not phenobarbital, significantly increased the time from falling asleep to the first rem period and significantly decreased the percentage of rem sleep. The subjects had less rem time on phenobarbital than on placebo, but this effect of phenobarbital did not reach statistical significance. Both drugs increased the percentage of stage 4 sleep. The duration of the first rem period was not affected by either agent. Feinberg (1969) found that phenobarbital, 200 mg, significantly decreased rem percentage. Baekeland (1967) studied the effect of pentobarbital on fifteen college students. Drug administration nights were one week apart. Pentobarbital decreased rem percentage, the number of awakenings during the night, the number of body movements, and the rem latency. The increase in nonrem sleep was distributed among the nonrem sleep stages. Hartmann (1968) studied the effect of pentobarbital and other drugs on ten young volunteers sleeping one night per week in the laboratory. The pentobarbital increased total sleep time, decreased rem percentage, and also decreased the time from the beginning of recording to the onset of sleep with the drug given thirty minutes prior to time of retiring. Williams and Agnew (1969) found pentobarbital to decrease rem and increase stage 2 sleep in a study which separated drug nights by only one drug-free night sleeping at home. Oswald and Priest (1965) in a longitudinal study recorded the sleep of two men for a number of consecutive nights. After five baseline nights the subjects took 400 mg of amylobarbitone nightly for nine nights. The rem percentage dropped for the first few nights but then rose toward normal. The dose of amylobarbitone was increased to 600 mg and given nightly for another nine consecutive nights. This increased dose again decreased rem percentage, but this decrease again proved transient. After abrupt drug withdrawal a marked increase of rem percentage occurred, accompanied by rem occurring earlier in the night. Some increase of rem in the early hours of the night or decreased latency to the first rem period continued for up to five weeks after only eighteen nights on the drug. Evans and Lewis (1968) replicated this study and found that chlorpromazine blocked the rem rebound. Lester and his co-workers (1968) reported that secobarbital, 200 mg, had no effect on rem sleep; the drug increased delta sleep in the first half of the night, but in the second half of the night less delta sleep occurred following administration of secobarbital than following administration of placebo. Haider (1969) reported that amylobarbitone, 200 mg in six normal volunteers, decreased rem sleep. The concomitant increase in nonrem was mainly in nonrem stage 2. This study was replicated by Haider and Oswald (1971). A combination of quinalbarbital, 100 mg, and amylobarbital, 100 mg, can decrease the percentage of the total sleep time spent in the rem state (Davison et al., 1970). Kales et al. (1970f) also described the rem suppressant and rem rebound effects of pentobarbital, 100 mg in four volunteers.

These results, deriving from both double-blind alternation and longitudinal experimental design, show conclusively that the barbiturates decrease rem percentage, that prolonged use of barbiturates causes a loss of this rem suppressant effect, and that drug withdrawal after chronic use produces a rem rebound.

ALCOHOL

Alcohol is the most commonly used psychoactive agent in Western civilization. No one can accurately estimate how many have crossed the wavy line between heavy social drinking and chronic alcoholism, but more people are addicted to alcohol than to all other psychoactive agents combined.

Gresham and his co-workers (1963) administered alcohol to seven medical students at a dose of 1 gm/kg of body weight, approximately the equivalent of six ounces of 100-proof whiskey. Because of its taste and smell, alcohol cannot be given in a double-blind manner. During each of three baseline nights the subjects drank orange juice, while on the two experimental nights alcohol or caffeine was alternately administered mixed in orange juice. Only the first 300 minutes of each night's total sleep time was reported. Alcohol caused a decrease from 71,38,46,106,86,73,61 minutes of rem on the average baseline night for each subject to 28,40,28,49,69,65,43 minutes respectively on the alcohol night. Not only is there great individual variation in percentage rem on baseline nights, but there is also great individual variation in response to alcohol. Yules et al. (1966) gave the same dose of alcohol in the same manner to three graduate students. Four baseline nights with orange juice in each subject gave a mean rem percentage of 24, 26, and 31 percent. Alcohol on the first night decreased these percentages to 19, 21, and 25 respectively. In the first half of the night this effect was more marked with decreases from 20, 13, and 20 percent to 14, 9, and 8. With continued administration of this same dose of alcohol every night for five nights, the percentage of rem returned toward the baseline values. The fourth alcohol night showed values of 29, 20, and 25. On the fifth alcohol night rem percentage rose above baseline to 28, 38, and 50. Upon stopping alcohol, rem percentages were above baseline values, being 38, 25, and 37 on the first post-alcohol night. In a later paper Yules et al. (1967) reported that the decrease in rem was made up for in the total sleep time by increases in nonrem stage 4. The rem latency, which is the time from the onset of sleep to the onset of the first rem period, was not affected in this experimental design either by alcohol or by alcohol withdrawal. Knowles et al. (1968) studied 3.5 oz or 6.0 oz of alcohol in one subject, who was one of the authors, over a number of nights. The lower of these doses did not change overall rem percentage, being 20.6 on the average of five baseline nights and 21.0 on four alcohol nights. By breaking up the night into halves, however, a marked inhibition of rem sleep appeared during the first half, being decreased from an average baseline value of 11.2 percent to 0 percent on two alcohol nights and an average of 2.0 percent on two later alcohol nights. A concomitant increase in rem percentage occurred in the second halves of these nights. Since length of sleep was not controlled, this latter finding could be related to the subject sleeping longer in the mornings following alcohol ingestion. On the larger dose of 6.0 oz of alcohol there was a decrease of overall rem percentage from 20.6 percent to 13.0 percent as the average of two high-dose alcohol nights and 15.0 percent on two other nights. A rebound effect on the nights following alcohol withdrawal was also suggested, particularly in the data from the first half of the night, but the exact numbers were not reported. Greenberg and Pearlman (1967) studied three subjects with varying doses of alcohol. One subject had no baseline record, but those who did showed a decrease in minutes and in percentage of rem on the first alcohol night. Steady increases in alcohol dosage prevented the tolerance reported by Yules et al. (1966), and the rem percentage remained relatively low. They also studied patients during alcohol withdrawal, including five subjects with delirium tremens. These five were sometimes continuously awake during D.T.s, but when they slept they had a high percentage of rem sleep. One patient who was recorded prior to the onset of D.T.s had 300 minutes of rem sleep, the highest rem time and rem percentage ever recorded. Gross et al. (1966) studied four alcoholic patients in alcohol withdrawal. During all-night recording the first night in the hospital two of these patients had no sleep whatsoever, but the two who slept showed a high percentage of rem, being 91 minutes of rem out of 91 minutes of sleep in one case and 185 minutes of rem out of 395 minutes of sleep in the other. Johnson and his co-workers (1970) also reported markedly elevated rem percentages during alcohol withdrawal. Mello and Mendelson (1970) found that long-term alcohol consumption in alcoholics caused an increased total sleep time and a marked fragmentation of the circadian sleep rhythm so that sleep was obtained in several naps, occurring both at night and in the daytime. The fragmentation of sleep into naps also occurred during alcohol withdrawal. Othmer and his colleagues (1970) have suggested that these naps may contain large amounts of rem sleep; they may even begin with sleep onset rem. Mello and Mendelson (1970) also noted that delirium tremens could occur without an antecedent or concurrent state of insomnia.

In summary, alcohol, like the barbiturates, increases total sleep time and decreases rem percentage. Withdrawal of alcohol from a person taking it for several days results in a pronounced rem rebound. This rem rebound is greater following alcohol withdrawal than following withdrawal of barbiturates or any other drug. The hallucinatory experiences of delirium tremens may be related to the underlying physiology of the rem state.

OTHER DRUGS

From a review of the studies summarized in Table XIII, one might formulate the general pharmacologic rule that most chemical agents which affect sleep depress the rem state. A few drugs such as reserpine, LSD, tryptophan, and 5-hydroxytryptophan facilitate the rem state in man as evidenced by an increase in rem percentage for the whole night or the first portion of the night, a decrease in rem latency, and a lengthening of the first or second rem periods. Most of these rem facilitating agents interact with brain serotonin. Of the many drugs which depress rem, most lose this rem suppression with chronic administration. This tolerance is probably due to internal brain homeostatic mechanisms which recognize the presence of rem suppression and adjust the rem generation mechanism. Withdrawal of drugs which suppress rem after the establishment of this tolerance causes a disturbed sleep characterized by a high percentage of rem sleep. This rem rebound may be "the result of the now unopposed compensatory process" (Feinberg and Evarts, 1969).

The monoamine oxidase inhibitor phenelzine can completely abolish the rem state. A dose of 60 mg has little or no effect the first night it is given. With chronic use of this agent, however, the rem percentage gradually falls until it reaches zero. Phenelzine, 60 mg, takes two to three weeks to abolish rem; a dose of 90 mg decreases rem to zero in a few days. This rem abolition can continue as long as the drug is administered, up to several weeks at least. Despite this lack of tolerance, abrupt discontinuance of phenelzine produces a clear and marked withdrawal rem overshoot. A dose of 45 mg of phenelzine decreases but does not abolish rem sleep; 30 mg has no effect. Yet if phenelzine in a dose of 60 to 90 mg has abolished rem, and if this dose is dropped to 30 mg, no rem rebound occurs. If then after several days the 30 mg dose is discontinued, the typical withdrawal rem rebound occurs (Akindele et al., 1970; Wyatt et al., 1971b).

One might suspect that all those drugs abused by modern society should have a similar effect on sleep. This, however, is not the case. LSD tends to increase the percentage of sleep spent in the rem type of sleep (Muzio et al., 1966; Green, 1965, 1969). Amphetamines decrease rem percentage and also decrease total sleep time (Rechtschaffen and Maron, 1964; Baekeland, 1967). Addicting substances which decrease rem percentage while tending to increase total sleep time include alcohol, barbiturates, morphine (Kay et al., 1969), and heroin (Lewis et al., 1970). Amphetamines, narcotics, barbiturates, and alcohol lose the rem-depressing effect with chronic administration and show a rem rebound following withdrawal. The decreasing effect with chronic use is, of course, physiologic tolerance, while the rem rebound is a physiologic withdrawal effect. A single dose of tetrahydrocannabinol, the active ingredient of marihuana, depresses rem sleep (Pivik et al., 1972), but no longitudinal study of the effect of marihuana on sleep has yet appeared. One would certainly like to see the results of such a study before joining Pillard (1970), Grinspoon (1971), and other drug experts in concluding that marihuana does not produce physiologic tolerance or any physiologic effects when withdrawn. The official statement of the World Health Organization Expert Committee on Drug Dependence (1969) that marihuana shows "little or no development of tolerance" may seem premature if further study shows an effect of the chronic use of marihuana and marihuana withdrawal on polygraphic sleep.

Pharmacologic studies utilizing the new methods of all-night polygraphy have given a new dimension to psychopharmacology. This chapter has reviewed some of the reasons why many of these studies are difficult and a few impossible to interpret. From the many different approaches to this type of research two basic strategies emerge:

1. The double-blind alternation strategy records the direct and immediate effect of a drug on sleep, free of any subconscious bias of the investigator.

2. The longitudinal study measures the chronic as well as the immediate effect of a pharmacologic agent and also permits the analysis of drug withdrawal.

Despite variability in strategy and procedure, studies with barbiturates and with alcohol show clear and reproducible effects on sleep. These agents decrease the percentage of sleep spent in the rem stage.

With chronic use, they lose this effect. When abruptly withdrawn after chronic use, both barbiturates and alcohol produce a rem rebound. Many other drugs have similar effects. The clinical use of sleeping pills is discussed in the next chapter.

Chapter 8

SLEEP DISORDERS

Sleep and watchfulness, both of them, when immoderate constitute disease.

HIPPOCRATES, *Aphorisms*

NARCOLEPSY AND HYPERSOMNIA

MODERN sleep research has helped to clarify the confusing disorder known as narcolepsy. Patients carrying this label range from the sleepy medical student to Dickens' character Joe the Fat Boy. Polygraphic studies have suggested that people who suffer attacks of an overwhelming desire for daytime sleep should be separated into two categories. A minority of these patients suffer from a specific disorder referred to as essential, primary, or true narcolepsy or Gelineau's syndrome. The fully developed form of the disorder presents the narcoleptic tetrad: sleep attacks, cataplexy (sudden weakness), hypnogogic hallucinations (vivid mentation at nocturnal sleep onset), and sleep paralysis (the feeling during or following sleep that one cannot move). In these patients, the sleep attack is an attack of the rem type of sleep. Nocturnal sleep is abnormal because it begins with a rem period. This entity is to be differentiated from the other category of daytime somnolence. This diverse group of disorders contains patients suffering generalized somnolence due to psychiatric disorder or brain dysfunction due to systemic or neurologic disease. The daytime sleep in these patients consists mainly of nonrem sleep. Many refer to this group of disorders as symptomatic, secondary, or pseudonarcolepsy or hypersomnia.

Future research may show true narcolepsy to be a syndrome, a pathologic reaction of the neural sleep mechanism to many inciting agents. At our present state of knowledge, however, it is best, I think, to consider true narcolepsy as a specific disease entity with specific, though unknown, underlying neuropathology and a characteristic natural history in order to facilitate the differentiation of this sleep

117

problem from the morass of confusing hypersomnias. The sleep attack of true narcolepsy is an overwhelming tiredness; but after the brief sleep is over, the patient feels refreshed. Early EEG studies described electrical rhythms characteristic of light drowsiness during the sleep attack of true narcolepsy (Daly and Yoss, 1957; Smith, 1959; Bulow and Ingvar, 1963). Polygraphic studies with recording of eye movements and chin EMG have shown that this attack is actually an attack of the rem type of sleep (Hishikawa and Kaneko, 1965; Dement et al., 1966; Roth et al., 1969). Twenty-four-hour recordings show that these rem attacks tend to occur at regular periods during the day (Passouant et al., 1968). The nocturnal sleep of narcoleptic patients is also abnormal; rem sleep occurs immediately after sleep onset rather than after one or two hours of the nonrem type of sleep (Rechtschaffen et al., 1963; Passouant et al., 1968). This probably explains the vivid mentation at sleep onset, the hypnogogic hallucinations. Similarly, the sleep paralysis occurs following a rem period (Suzuki, 1966; Hishikawa et al., 1965, 1968; Nan'no et al., 1970). In cataplexy, the patient's knees give way and he falls to the ground. Emotional events, particularly laughter or some type of internal conflict, triggers cataplectic attacks. "If I must laugh or be where there is much excitement," said one patient (recorded by Kamman, 1929), "I must place my hands on some object that will hold my weight. My strength leaves me until I haven't the strength of a tiny babe. At first my knees double up and I fall. From there the weakness spreads to my neck and my head falls forward or sideways." Some workers think that cataplexy is also a sudden attack of rem sleep, with the sleep terminated by the sudden shock of striking the ground (Scollo-Lavizzari, 1970). Actually, the first narcoleptic attack observed by physicians demonstrated the relationship of cataplexy, sleep attack, and sleep paralysis, as reported by S.A.K. Wilson (1928):

> While I was occupied with another patient, E.C. was sitting behind me and, as afterwards appeared, was endeavoring to keep himself from falling asleep. (This is the description of an irresistible sleep attack). Suddenly I heard a slight groaning sound coming from him, and at once looking around I saw his head nodding gently on his chest as he sank forward into a bent position and a moment or two later slid or slithered off the chair on the floor. (This may be cataplexy.) The arms were by the side and the fingers semiflexed; the eyes were closed. Lift-

ing the arms I found them absolutely atonic and flaccid; when let go they fell like lumps of lead by the side. The legs similarly were absolutely atonic, sprawling out on the floor. Lifting the eyelids I observed that the pupils reacted to light slightly but definitely, while the eyelid muscles were so toneless that little or no reflex contraction took place on my touching the cornea. Testing the knee-jerks I found them completely abolished on both sides. In the meantime Dr. (Macdonald) Critchley had hurriedly taken off the patient's shoe and sock on the left side, and testing the plantar reflex obtained a slight but definite extensor response, which he demonstrated to me and which I corroborated.

Just as we were finishing this rapid examination the patient suddenly said, "I'm all right, sir," in his ordinary voice, and with a faint smile. Muscular power came back; he moved his limbs, got on to the chair, and told us he had been conscious the whole time. He described what we had done, from lifting the eyelids to scratching the sole of the left foot. (Apparently this was sleep paralysis.) The duration of the whole attack was from sixty to ninety seconds. Testing his knee-jerks again, I found them active, even brisk on both sides, two minutes after he had recovered. So far as I am aware this is the first time a neurological examination of a patient in the cataplectic state has been recorded.

True narcolepsy is a characteristic disorder of sleep whose exact etiology and pathogenesis remain a mystery wrapped in the enigma of sleep itself. In some patients, additional symptoms appear including psychiatric disorders such as chronic anxiety, depression, and schizophrenia as well as fugue states and periods of amnesia (Pond, 1952; Ganado, 1958; Sours, 1963). Cases of true narcolepsy with unusual reaction to alcohol (Goodwin et al., 1970) or with the sensation of looking at color television while actually watching a black and white set (McCrary and Smith, 1967) have been reported. This disorder usually begins in adolescence or young adulthood; it continues throughout life but is generally thought to improve in later years. The improvement may be an adjustment of life style to fit the illness rather than any real change in the underlying disease process. Many stimulant and antidepressant medications have been used in the treatment of true narcolepsy, but nothing replaces an understanding discussion with the patient and his family about the illness and ways they can adjust themselves to it. An example of environmental treatment is given by Parker (1956). A young teacher suffered greatly from true narcolepsy, frequently falling asleep while driving to and from his school. By arranging to nap along the road and by having a bed available at the school where he could sleep off these brief attacks, the man became totally adjusted to his affliction. In certain intractable cases the rem-blocking monoamine oxidase inhibiter phenelzine can be used (Wyatt et al., 1971a).

Pseudonarcolepsy is frequently associated with underlying brain disease; true narcolepsy but rarely. Narcolepsy with cataplexy has been described associated with neurologic disorders including multiple sclerosis (Ekbom, 1966), frontal lobe meningioma (Hunter et al., 1968), and epidemic encephalitis (Kamman, 1929). Symonds (1954) described a patient with cataplexy alone who had signs and symptoms of syringomyelia. This patient might also have had syringobulbia with destruction of brain stem sleep-related structures. Hobson (1970) briefly described a fifty-four-year-old man with brief but very frequent rem sleep attacks. At postmortem examination, neuronal loss, astrocytosis, and demyelination were seen throughout the central nervous system, but the most severe involvement was in the pontine tegmentum.

Many medical, neurologic, and psychiatric conditions interfere with the sleep mechanism to cause episodic or nonepisodic diurnal sleepiness. These sleep attacks consist mainly of nonrem sleep. Nocturnal sleep usually does not begin with a rem period in this diverse group of patients suffering from hypersomnia. This type of sleep disorder can occur in patients with brain tumors, encephalitis, drug-induced acute encephalopathy, head trauma, and cerebrovascular disease (Hurwitz et al., 1959). African trypanosomiasis, the original sleeping sickness, is associated with abnormalities of nonrem sleep (Schwartz and Escande, 1970). Periods of somnolence and overeating lasting days to weeks separated by periods of normality form the Kleine-Levin syndrome (Levin, 1936; Garland et al., 1965; Duffy and Davison, 1968; Persson et al., 1969). Oswald (1969) doubts the existence of this syndrome as a specific entity. The waking EEG in the periods of normal behavior in these patients is entirely normal while during an attack slow activity is prominent (Elian and Bornstein, 1969; Thacore et al., 1969). Sleepiness is the major symptom of the Pickwickian syndrome. Patients with extreme obesity sometimes have such a low tidal volume that, despite an increased respiratory rate, reduced alveolar ventilation results in hypoxemia and increased carbon dioxide retention (Cayler et al., 1961). We do not know which, if either, of these respiratory abnormalities produces hypersomnia. Some clinicians feel that a basic underlying neurologic disorder, probably involving the hypothalamus, produces sleepiness and obesity due to insatiable hunger in some Pickwickian patients. The EEG during periods of sleep in these obese patients shows slow waves characteristic of nonrem sleep (Drachman and Gummit, 1962; Jung and Kuhlo, 1965). This disorder is called the Pickwickian syndrome after the famous character in Charles Dickens' *Pickwick Papers:*

> "Damn that boy," said the old gentleman, "he gone to sleep again."
> "Very extraordinary boy, that," said Mr. Pickwick, "does he always sleep in this way?"
> "Sleep!" said the old gentleman, "he's always asleep. Goes on errands fast asleep, and snores as he waits at table."
> "How very odd!" said Mr. Pickwick.
> "Ah! Odd indeed," returned the old gentleman; "I'm proud of that boy—wouldn't part with him on any account—damn, he's a natural curiosity! Here, Joe, Joe, take these things away, and open another bottle—d'ye hear?"
> The fat boy rose, opened his eyes, swallowed the huge piece of pie he had been in the act of masticating when he last fell asleep and slowly obeyed his master's orders.

Of course, there are a large number of people who sleep under boring conditions, such as a lecture. Stossel (1970) for example, studied medical students during morning lectures. He defined a student as sleeping if his eyes were shut for at least three minutes; 24 percent of students slept at some time during the average lecture. During the worst lectures over half the students fell asleep. Pauker (1970) actually reported that the loss of muscle tone during medical lectures can come on so quickly that cervical muscle spasm can result from "whiplash"-like injury. Of course, these students were not studied polygraphically, but daytime EEGs from patients who complain of diurnal sleepiness alone, without associated symptoms such as cataplexy, have shown that the sleep attacks are actually periods of nonrem sleep (Dement et al., 1966; Roth et al., 1969). Nocturnal sleep from these patients begins with a nonrem period as does normal sleep; however, these individuals may have cyclic periods of rem and nonrem sleep into the late morning hours (Rechtschaffen and Roth, 1969). Globus (1969) has suggested that the abnormally large amounts of sleep in some late risers may produce psychiatric symptoms and feelings of lethargy, sometimes called the "blah" syndrome. The reverse is just as likely; persons suffering psychiatric symptoms may sleep late as a defense against facing the world (Hartmann et al., 1971).

Table XIV reviews some of the differential points between narcolepsy and hypersomnia, between true narcolepsy and pseudonarcolepsy. The importance of this differentiation was reemphasized to me quite recently. I was in my office, working on Chapter 3 of this book, when I was interrupted by a call to see a "narcoleptic" who was being treated with methylphenidate, 10 mg, three times a day.

> The patient was a 64-year-old black woman who had been suffering diurnal sleepiness for about one or two years. The disease had, according to the patient's husband, began insidiously. Daytime naps and occasional nocturnal restlessness progressed to lethargy, then almost continuous somnolence. The patient now slept all the time except when roused for meals. There was no history of cataplexy, sleep paralysis, or hypnogogic hallucinations. When I examined the patient she appeared to be sleeping soundly. When vigorously roused by shaking she would sleepily look about and answer a simple question or two before slipping back to sleep. The patient had bilateral optic atrophy and generalized hyperreflexia without any other abnormal physical findings. The sense of smell was not tested. The skull x-ray was interpreted as normal; the sella turcica was not enlarged. An electroencephalogram showed generalized slow activity without any sleep spindles (Fig. 15). Although the patient had noticed polyuria and polydipsia, time did not permit a neuroendocrine evaluation. The cerebral angiograms revealed a suprasellar mass which was removed surgically (Fig. 16). The mass involved the optic nerves and chiasm, the hypothalamus, the preoptic area and the orbital surface of both frontal lobes. Histologic evaluation of the mass revealed it to be a suprasellar chromophobe adenoma. Unfortunately bleeding occurred from both anterior cerebral arteries during the operation and the patient died in the immediate postoperative period. This patient had hypersomnolence as a symptom of a fatal brain tumor; she did not have true narcolepsy.

In summary, patients with daytime sleep attacks can be divided into two groups. A small but fairly homogeneous group suffers from sleep attacks associated with cataplexy, sleep paralysis, and hypnogogic hallucinations. Polygraphic studies have shown that the sleep attack

TABLE XIV
DIFFERENTIATION OF NARCOLEPSY AND HYPERSOMNIA

	Narcolepsy	Hypersomnia
Synonyms:	True narcolepsy Narcolepsy with cataplexy Gelineau's syndrome	Pseudonarcolepsy Symptomatic narcolepsy
Etiology:	Unknown in the vast majority of cases; rarely associated with a structural CNS lesion.	Many psychiatric, medical, and neurological causes.
Sleep attacks:	Episodic, overpowering, usually a brief sleep refreshes. Usually rem sleep.	Sleepiness may be episodic or continual; frequently sleep does not refresh. Usually nonrem sleep.
Other symptoms:	Cataplexy, sleep paralysis, hynogogic hallucinations.	None or other symptoms associated with underlying lesion.
Nocturnal sleep:	May or may not be disturbed; sleep onset rem periods.	Sometimes disturbed by loss of circadian sleep-waking rhythm; sometimes somnolence is continuous day and night.
Treatment:	Directed at acceptance of illness; pharmacologic treatment is secondary.	Directed at underlying cause.

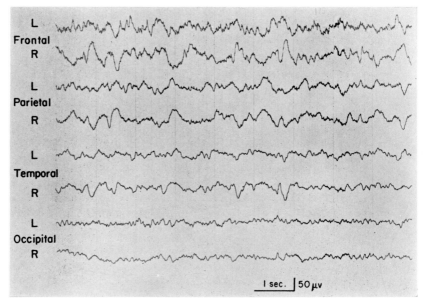

Figure 15. The clinical EEG shows generalized slow activity of greater amplitude on the right and anteriorly, without sleep spindles.

in these individuals is an attack of rem sleep, and the nocturnal sleep of these patients begins with a rem period. A large heterogeneous group of people have nonrem sleep periods during the day with the normal appearance of a nonrem period to intiate nocturnal sleep. This latter group includes normal people who sleep during boring periods such as lectures, patients with Pickwickian syndrome or Kleine-Levin syndrome, and a larger number of people with various types of brain pathology.

INSOMNIA

When faced with a patient complaining of insomnia, the physician considers that this symptom may represent underlying medical or psychiatric illness: the insomnia of alcohol or drug withdrawal, the frequent awakenings of cardiac disease, the difficulty falling asleep in patients enduring pain, the early morning awakening of depression. These problems will be considered in the next chapter. This section examines the type of insomnia suffered by otherwise healthy people.

Everyone has occasional difficulty falling asleep, particularly on

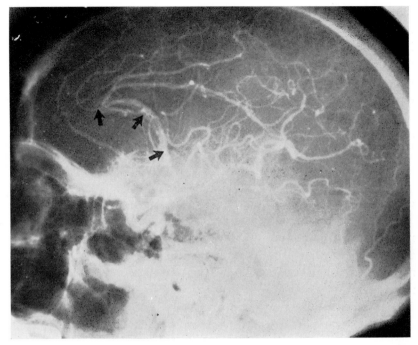

Figure 16. The right carotid arteriogram. A large hypothalamic and frontal lobe mass elevates the right anterior cerebral artery.

nights following a traumatic occurrence such as a minor auto accident or on nights preceding an anticipated event, either a happy event like a marriage or a dreaded event like a marriage. With all his worries it is not surprising that Job suffered insomnia:

> When I lie down I say, when shall I arise and the night be gone?
> And I am full of tossings to and fro unto the dawning of the day
>
> JOB 7:4

In the United States about 20 percent of young, healthy people complain of chronic difficulty falling asleep; this insomnia is more common in women than in men (Raybin and Detre, 1969). Monroe (1967) recorded all-night electroencephalography in individuals who described themselves as poor sleepers. These people, as compared to a group of good sleepers, had greater sleep latency, more awakenings, a higher percentage of nonrem stage 2, and shorter rem periods giving an overall decreased rem percentage. Slow wave sleep was the same in the two groups. Normal subjects have less rem and increased sleep latency on the first night than on later nights in the sleep laboratory probably due to anxiety and uncertainty about the experimental equipment and the nature of the experiment. Greenberg (1967) has described individuals who frequently awaken from rem periods because of fearful elements occurring in the ongoing rem mentation. One cannot necessarily equate decreased sleep time with insomnia, as shown by the two normal, active men discussed in Chapter 1 who usually sleep only three hours per night; their sleep contains large amounts of nonrem stages 3 and 4 and a normal percentage, but of course a decreased total amount, of rem sleep.

In a manner similar to the treatment of hiccups, an astronomical number of suggestions have been offered to aid one in falling asleep rapidly. Counting sheep is the classic example. One of the better methods is to go through a specific and unchanging routine each night before bed and once in bed never to think about events planned for the following day. Special training during wakefulness to develop the ability to relax tense muscles has been suggested (Kahn et al., 1968). Storms and Nisbett (1970) recommend the use of placebos which the patient is told is a stimulant, not a sedative. The traditional medical approach to insomnia is the use of sedatives.

In the last century, Lyman (1885) recommended the following drugs for the treatment of insomnia: digitalis, camphor, valerian, cannabis indica, belladonna, hyoscyamus, opium, paraldehyde, chloral hydrate, chloroform, ether, bromides, and alcohol. Today's list of sleep-producing medications is similar; only the names have changed. We still lack any real knowledge of how the herbs of the nineteenth century or the chemicals of the twentieth century aid sleep induction. The major advance in modern sleep pharmacology is the validation of the old clinical dictum against the chronic use of sleeping pills.

As discussed in the previous chapter, the most frequently prescribed hypnotics, the barbiturates, have consistent effects on sleep. To review, these drugs suppress rem sleep, lose this suppression with chronic administration, and produce rem rebound on withdrawal. Most other drugs used clinically as sleep-producing agents have similar effects. Meprobamate, alpha chloralose, nitrazepam, glutethimide (Doriden®), morphine, methyprylon (Nodudar®), as well as alcohol and scopolamine (present in many nonprescription sleeping potions) suppress rem sleep, and many of these agents cause a rem rebound when abruptly withdrawn after chronic administration (see Table XIII). Chloral hydrate and flurazepam (Dalmane®) at a dose of 30 mg have been studied by all-night polygraphy, and no effect on rem percentage has yet been demonstrated. At a dosage level of 60 mg, flurazepam suppresses rem. While one study showed methaqualone (Quaalude®) to have no effect on rem sleep, another laboratory showed that this agent at a dose of 300 mg lowers rem percentage, and that withdrawal after three consecutive nights produces an increase in rem percentage above baseline levels.

Should the physician prescribe a sleeping pill which suppresses rem in order to make the night seem subjectively more restful by decreasing the amount of emotional rem mentation? Recall the "deep and dreamless" sleep mentioned in Chapter 6. Preliminary studies have shown that mentation during rem sleep following hypnotics is less vivid than rem mentation on a night without the drug (Kales et al., 1969; Carroll et al., 1969). In certain medical conditions discussed in the next chapter, rem suppression is desirable. For simple insomnia, however, our present state of knowledge does not permit us to say whether the rem suppression produced by the single night use of a hypnotic is detrimental, desirable, or neutral. One thing we can declare, though, with incontrovertible certitude, is that the rem rebound following withdrawal of the chronic use of a drug is one of the commonest causes of sleep disturbance. This rem rebound is associated with difficulty falling asleep and with increased vividness of rem mentation progressing to terrifying nightmares (Oswald, 1968). Every physician has seen the patient who demands sleeping pills (Johnson and Clift, 1968; Franklin, 1969; Kane, 1970). "I just can't sleep without those pills." For that patient, the sleeping pills are not improving some underlying sleep disturbance; all they are doing is preventing the signs and symptoms of their own withdrawal.

The chronic use of a rem-suppressing hypnotic fulfills many criteria for iatrogenic addiction: the drug produces a tolerance and its withdrawal produces physiological withdrawal effects. While hypnotic medication may be very helpful for a single unusual night like the first night in the hospital, all-night polygraphic research suggests that these drugs should seldom be used chronically. It is the author's opinion that the promiscuous prescribing of sleep medications is the most common error in medicine. For single-night use, any of the sleep-producing drugs can be recommended save the barbiturates, which have a high suicide potential. Actually, the intelligent clinician was aware of the dangers of overdependence on sedatives prior to the development of all-night polygraphic studies:

> It is sensible to take a sedative on an overnight train or plane ride, or on the first night or two of a head cold. A sedative may be useful at the end of a long, arduous trip or after any form of prolonged excitement. The wise physician often prescribes a sedative for the patient in the early stages of an acute infection or in any state of acute discomfort. Wakefulness in such conditions serves no useful purpose. The underlying cause is known and temporary, and habituation to sedatives under these conditions need not be feared. The situation is quite different in neurotic insomnia, in which the cause is psychologic, unconscious, and chronic. . . . The patient's symptoms will recur, and more and different sedatives will be prescribed. What is worse, habituation to these drugs may come about, and the patient's neurotic complaint that his trouble is physical and not psychologic is aided and abetted. Here, one is faced with perhaps the commonest of iatrogenic disorders. (Solomon, 1956)

SLOW WAVE SLEEP DISORDERS

The classic sleep disorders of somnambulism, enuresis, and nocturnal terrors involve nonrem stages 3 and 4, slow wave sleep. Sleep talking also usually occurs in nonrem sleep, particularly stages 3 and 4, though an occasional unusual patient sleep talks mainly during the rem state (Arkin et al., 1970).

Sleepwalking usually begins in childhood. The sufferer awakens in the morning to see clothes scattered and other nocturnal activity for which he has no memory. Family members may see the patient walk about in his sleep, performing somewhat complicated acts like unlocking a door. When they address the sleepwalker, he may reply or he may mumble nonsense phrases. If he is forcibly awakened by shaking, the sleepwalker is disoriented and confused to a greater degree than one wakened from normal sleep. Since other family members may be sleepwalkers, frequently medical consultation is not obtained, and the incidence of this condition remains unknown. Bakin (1970) reports a 47 percent concordance for sleepwalking in monozygotic twins compared to 7 percent for dizygotic indicating a genetic component in this disorder. One might have predicted that the sleepwalking occurred during a rem period and was the "acting out of a dream." Several studies have shown, however, that sleepwalking always begins during nonrem stages 3 and 4 (Kales et al., 1966; Jacobson et al., 1965; Broughton, 1968). During the walking, the delta activity can be replaced by faster frequencies. After the attack the patient can awaken or can return to sleep, usually entering stage 2.

Nocturnal bedwetting in children past the age of 4 or 5 is abnormal. The psychologic problems which result from this involuntary bedwetting and from parents' and society's reaction to it can be serious, as described by a victim of this disorder, George Orwell (1952):

> I knew that bedwetting was (a) wicked and (b) outside my control. The second fact I was personally aware of, and the first I did not question. It was possible, therefore, to commit a sin without knowing you committed it, without wanting to commit it, and without being able to avoid it.

Nocturnal enuresis occurs during or following nonrem sleep (Finley, 1971). In adults particularly, slow wave sleep ends and a variable period characterized by an EEG containing alpha activity intervenes before the actual enuresis. This EEG picture, which is more akin to wakefulness than any sleep stage, is accompanied by behavioral sleep; the patient's eyes are closed and arousal is associated with transient disorientation (Schiff, 1965). Broughton (1968) recorded bladder pressure in enuretic children throughout the night and was able to measure small contractions of the detrusor muscle of the bladder. These occurred in enuretic children even on those nights when they suffered no bedwetting but did not occur in a group of normal children. Only during nonrem stages 3 and 4 did these detrusor contractions build up to such a level as to cause bladder emptying.

When a person complains of a bad dream, he probably has suffered unusually anxious rem mentation and has awakened from a rem period. The extremely severe nightmare, however, occurs during nonrem stage 4 sleep (Broughton, 1968; Fisher et al., 1970). The sleeper awakens screaming, with increased heart and respiratory rates. The sleeper may be unable to describe what type of sleep mental activity frightened him, or he may describe a sensation of choking or suffocating.

Drugs which decrease the percentage of stage 4 sleep have been recommended in the treatment of these slow wave sleep disorders (Kahn et al., 1970; Glick et al., 1971). Broughton (1968) postulates that the symptoms which interrupt slow wave sleep are due to dysfunction of arousal mechanisms. A real understanding of these disorders requires a more complete description of the autonomic and emotional concomitants of slow wave sleep in these patients and in normal persons.

Chapter 9

OTHER CLINICAL ASPECTS OF SLEEP

The sleeping patient is still a patient. His disease not only goes on
while he sleeps but indeed may progress in an entirely different fashion
from its progression during the waking state.

EUGENE ROBIN, 1958

GENERAL MEDICINE

OF all the general medical disorders, ischemic heart disease
most frequently causes sleep disturbance (Johns et al., 1970).
Karacan and his co-workers (1969) monitored the nocturnal sleep
of ten angina pectoris patients. The patients had only eighteen
minutes of nonrem stages 3 and 4; a group of ten age-matched
controls had forty-three minutes. When they awoke during the night,
the patients took longer to return to sleep than the control subjects.
The rem percentages were the same in both groups. All of these
changes could be the result of anxiety or might result from hemo-
dynamic adjustments to sleep or to the recumbent posture. Nowlin
and his colleagues (1965) reported that patients who awaken with
angina usually awaken from a rem period. Using all-night electro-
cardiography in addition to other polygraphic variables, they found
that cardiac arrhythmias occur much more frequently during rem
than during nonrem sleep.

Other diseases which have rem-associated exacerbations include
migraine headaches and duodenal ulcer. Dexter and Weitzman
(1970) reported three patients with nocturnal migraine and three with
cluster headaches who suffered severe headaches awakening them from
sleep. All-night polygraphic studies revealed that these headaches
began during a rem period. Armstrong et al. (1965) reported that
duodenal ulcer patients had increased gastric acid secretion during
rem but not during nonrem periods. This variation is gastric acid
secretion did not occur in control sleepers without duodenal ulcer

131

disease. Asthma attacks can begin in any sleep stage though they are less frequent in stage 4 than in other nonrem stages or than in rem sleep (Kales et al., 1970). Drugs which suppress rem sleep have been recommended for patients with ischemic heart disease, duodenal ulcer, or nocturnal migraine. As discussed at length previously, these drugs may be helpful in an acute situation such as the first days after a myocardial infarction, but most drugs cannot be used chronically because rem percentage will return to normal; one must beware of increased rem sleep and nightmares when the drug is withdrawn.

Sleep is disordered in uremia with frequent awakenings and decreased slow wave sleep (Passouant et al., 1970). Improvement in the uremia by dialysis returns sleep toward normal. Patients on maintenance hemodialysis at home, though, report that they sleep less on dialysis nights than on nights between dialysis treatments; their spouses sleep less on dialysis nights too (Daly and Hassal, 1970). Patients with hypothyroidism have a decreased amount of stage 4 sleep, increasing with thyroid treatment (Kales et al., 1967). Hypothyroid infants have a slower development of the spindles of stage 2 sleep than normal infants (Schultz et al., 1968). A single case of progeria has been studied by Rosenbloom et al. (1970). The sleep pattern was normal for the patient's age and did not resemble that seen in old age. Experimental fever can decrease rem and slow wave sleep time (Karacan et al., 1968b). Williams and Cartwright (1969) have studied five hypertensive women, recording blood pressure every two minutes throughout the night as well as electroencephalogram and eye movements. Though blood pressure did fall in the later part of the night, there was no difference between average blood pressure during rem and during nonrem sleep; it was high in both types of sleep. These hypertensive patients, however, had a variable blood pressure during all sleep stages unlike normal people whose blood pressure shows such variations only during rem sleep.

The sleep of alcoholics is deranged, associated with increased wakefulness and vivid dreams and nightmares (Johnson et al., 1970). All-night EEG studies of alcohol withdrawal have shown that the rem percentage may rise to 100 percent on the night before the onset of delirium tremens (see Chapter 7). Occasional rare patients have been reported who suffer hallucinations associated with a high rem percentage but without a history of alcoholism (Feinberg et al., 1965).

Pregnant women also have sleep derangements. All-night polygraphic studies have shown that during the last portion of gestation, the pregnant woman has difficulty falling asleep, frequent awakenings, and a marked reduction of slow wave sleep. There is some evidence that the sleep cycles of the mother and the fetus may be interrelated, presumably by humoral mechanisms (Petre-Quadens et al., 1967). After delivery, the new mother has very low rem percentage during nocturnal sleep (Karacan et al., 1968). Karacan and his co-workers (1969) have suggested that the low amount of rem sleep immediately pre- and post-partum could trigger a postpartum psychosis in a susceptible individual; in schizophrenia in remission, experimental rem deprivation does not cause a relapse (Vogel and Traub, 1968).

One cannot know if the abnormal sleep patterns of these patients represent specific disease pathophysiology or are only related to the emotional reaction of the patient to his illness and to the experimental situation. Particularly difficult to interpret is the decreased slow wave sleep one sees in a large number of conditions including pregnancy, depression, schizophrenia, hypothyroidism, epilepsy, ischemic heart disease, and many others.

Other suggestions for the clinical application of polygraphic sleep research include postoperative care of ophthalmologic patients and diagnosis of impotence. Kales, Adams, and Pearlman (1970a) point out that following some types of eye surgery, eye movements must be avoided while sutures heal. The use of drugs which suppress rem sleep might be important in the postoperative care of these patients. Karacan (1970) has suggested that the penile erection which accompanies rem periods may help differentiate psychologic from organic causes of the inability to obtain an erection during wakefulness.

CLINICAL NEUROLOGY

Organic brain lesions interfere with sleep patterns. Feinberg and his colleagues (1965b) recorded sleep patters in demented old people. Six patients with dementia probably due to extensive cerebrovascular disease had less total sleep time and a smaller rem percentage than a group of elderly people who were not demented. A patient with dementia associated with repeated episodes of subarachnoid hemorrhage had only 8 percent rem sleep. A patient with Korsakov's syndrome associated with alcoholism had a rem percentage of 13, not too far below the mean for his age group. Greenberg et al. (1968) found that patients developing the Korsakov syndrome had increased rem time while those individuals who had had the syndrome over one year had normal rem percentages. Since these authors studied individuals who had only been off alcohol for two weeks, it is possible that the increased rem percentage in the subacute group may have been related to the alcohol withdrawal state. The rem mentation in these individuals and in patients with short-term memory loss due to bilateral hippocampal destruction following encephalitis (Torda, 1969) lack day residue; the rem reports consist of single repetitive scenes related either to immediate needs such as hunger or to events from the distant past. Feldman (1971) reported a patient with paralysis below the eyes because of pontine destruction. This patient had several very brief rem periods totaling only 4 percent of the sleeping time. Adey and his co-workers (1968) found markedly decreased rem percentages in patients with quadraplegia due to destruction of the cervical spinal cord. These studies suggest that in man neural elements in the caudal brain stem and perhaps within the cervical spinal cord facilitate rem sleep. Extended polygraphic recordings in patients with coma due to head trauma have shown that the appearance of regular sleep cycles is a favorable prognostic sign (Passouant et al., 1965; Bergamasco et al., 1968). Less severe head injuries may produce sleep characterized by a decrease of stage 4 and a concomitant increase in stage 2 (Lenard and Penningstorff, 1970). Newborn infants suffering perinatal anoxia lose normal alternation of the infant sleep cycles (Dreyfus-Brisac and Monod, 1970). Normal sleep patterns are present in hyperactive children carrying the diagnosis of hyperkinetic syndrome due to minimal brain dysfunction (Small et al., 1971).

In addition to modifying sleep stage percentages, organic brain lesions in man can interfere with the phasic components of sleep. As a general rule, lesions which abolish a certain type of voluntary eye movement during waking prevent the same type of eye movements from occurring during rem sleep. Appenzeller and Fischer (1968) compared disorders of eye movements during wakefulness with eye movements during the rem stage of sleep. A patient unable to look to the left during wakefulness because of a right frontal hemisphere lesion affecting the "frontal gaze center" had no eye movements to the left during rem periods. A patient with progressive supranuclear palsy had absence during wakefulness of all eye movements except the ability to look conjugately downward. During rem periods only downward eye movements occurred. A patient with a hemorrhage in the left pons had, during wakefulness, inability to look to the left, presumably because of involvement of the "pontine gaze center," a clinical construct without anatomical counterpart. Similarly, during rem periods, the individual showed eye movements to the right but not to the left. Appenzeller and Fischer (1968) also reported absent eye movements during rem periods in several patients with chronic Wernicke's disease or Korsakov's syndrome associated with alcoholism. They hypothesized that this absence of eye movements was due to involvement of vestibular nuclei in Wernicke-Korsakov disorder. Jacobs et al. (1971b) studied five patients with upward gaze paralysis during waking. Two of these patients had pinealomas. As the patients fell into nonrem sleep their eyes turned upward, as in normal persons. During rem periods, no upward eye movements occurred. In patients with congenital nystagmus, the nystagmoid eye movements disappear as the person falls asleep, and the eye movements of rem sleep are free of nystagmus (Arkin et al., 1966). Starr (1967) reported that sleep patterns were normal in Huntington's chorea except that no eye movements occurred in otherwise normal rem periods.

In an extensive study of nonrem sleep in patients with brain tumors, Daly (1968) reported that those patients who had focal slow waves in the waking EEG due to a hemispheric tumor had persistence of this slow wave focus during all stages of nonrem sleep though its presence was largely obscured during stages 3 and 4 by generalized slow activity. Reduced sleep spindles frequently occurred ipsilateral to the hemispheric lesion. In those patients with diffuse rhythmic slow waves during wakefulness due to midline or infratentorial tumors, on the other hand, the appearance of sleep tended to eliminate the abnormal rhythm. Rem sleep was not studied. Daly closed with the interesting predicition that "systematic prospective studies which combine precise anatomical localization with meticulous observations of both reactivity and the abnormal waking and sleeping rhythms will disclose unexpected vistas." In patients with increased intracranial pressure, transient further increases in pressure may produce bursts of slow waves in the EEG during nonrem sleep, but not during waking or the rem state (Cooper and Hulme, 1969).

Charcot, the father of modern clinical neurology, thought that

Parkinson's disease or paralysis agitans was a psychogenic disorder because the tremor so characteristic of this malady disappeared during
sleep. Stern and co-workers (1968) performed all-night recording and
found that the parkinsonian tremor which disappeared when the
patient fell asleep, did not reappear in any sleep stage. The only
exceptions to this rule were very rare bursts of typical parkinsonian
pill rolling tremor in a few rem periods and even fewer nonrem stage
2 periods. Those occasions of tremor during nonrem stage 2 always
occurred within five minutes of a rem period, either before or after.
On those occasions when tremor occurred it was usually, but not
always, accompanied by a body movement. The tremor during rem
sleep always occurred simultaneously with a burst of rapid eye movements. During stage 2 the tremor was not related to sleep spindle
activity. Friedlander (1952) had previously noted the lack of correlation between sleep spindles and tremor. Kales and his co-workers
(1971) found six parkinsonian patients to have more difficulty falling
and staying asleep than a control group consisting of the patient's
spouses. Rem percentage was normal in the parkinsonian individuals.
By dividing patients with Parkinson's disease into clinical categories,
Traczynska et al. (1969) found that those patients with severe rigidity
had a decreased rem percentage.

An interesting neurological condition which has not been studied
with all-night polygraphic techniques is the occurrence of peripheral
nerve pain at night, either associated with a definite peripheral nerve
disorder such as carpal tunnel syndrome or a more diffuse acropar-
esthesia of no specific peripheral nerve (Hassin, 1951). Presumably,
in most people some type of reflex causes body movement when a nerve
is becoming ischemic due to prolonged pressure. In some conditions
this reflex type of arousal may be disturbed. Patients in coma, of
course, have total abolition of this reflex and must be protected from
pressure palsies. Pressure palsy is so common following severe alcoholic
intoxication that it is referred to among heavy drinkers as "Saturday
night palsy."

MENTAL RETARDATION

Mental retardation is, of course, a syndrome or a condition, not a
specific disease entity. Many cases of MR are caused by perinatal
factors: placenta previa, maternal toxemia, hyperbilirubinemia with

subsequent kernicterus, anoxia due to difficult labor. The majority of the mentally retarded never have a direct cause identified. Some cases of mild mental retardation are due to deprivation of interacting environmental stimuli during key times of brain development. Other cases of MR have a specific environmental cause such as lead poisoning, hydrocephalus, or meningoencephalitis. A very small minority have a distinct hereditary syndrome either due to an absent enzyme (example: PKU), to an abnormal chromosome (example: mongolism), or to unknown genetic mechanisms (example: myotonic dystrophy). The attempt to study the "average" mentally retarded, then, can never be totally successful.

This difficulty occurs in sleep research; for example, Petre-Quadens and Jouvet (1966) studied the sleep of forty-three mental retardates and compared these with twenty-eight normals. The mentally retarded had an average of 15.7 percent of their sleeping time occupied by rem sleep while the control group had an average rem percentage of 21.9. A few of the MR individuals, however, had very high rem percentages, up to almost 40 percent of the sleeping time. In a later communication, Petre-Quadens and Jouvet (1967) broke down these results by cause of the MR. While they gave no specific numbers, they stated that mongols had a normal percentage of rem sleep but had a longer total sleeping time with an increase of nonrem stage 4. In addition, the mongols showed periods of apparent sleep with an EEG of low voltage but without eye movements. The patients with MR of unknown etiology had a decreased percentage of rem sleep. The individuals with cystinuria and PKU showed a decrease in total sleeping time, particularly marked in the PKU patients. These two disorders were associated with a decreased rem percentage. Fewer eye movements occurred during the rem sleep of these retarded children than during the rem sleep of normal children of the same age (Petre-Quadens and de Lee, 1970). Goldie and his co-workers (1968) studied the sleep patterns of five newborn mongols during daytime. They reported that the average duration of each nonrem period was abnormally long, being 23.7 minutes in the mongols compared to 13.6 minutes in control normal newborns. The sleep of these retarded newborns was characterized by an increased period of transition from rem to nonrem sleep periods, frequent side-to-side head movements during nonrem, and qualitative changes in the EEG recording during nonrem sleep. This data from mongol neonates is not directly comparable to the results of Petre-Quadens and Jouvet (1967) in older mongol children. By dividing mongol children into groups according to the severity of the mental retardation, Castaldo (1968) found that the more severely affected had less rem time and a longer rem latency than the mildly retarded mongols. Karacan and his co-workers (1966) reported the sleep patterns in twelve infants and children with Tay-Sachs disease; diagnosis in nine of these cases was made by histologic examination of brain tissue. In Tay-Sachs patients of one to two years of age, the mean sleeping time in a 24-hour period was 26 percent with only a quarter of this time spent in rem sleep. Patients between ages two and three had 41 percent sleep with 31 percent of this time spent in the rem stage of sleep. Two older individuals had no discernable rem sleep and had 53 percent of a 24-hour period spent in sleep as determined by behavioral observations; waking EEG was so abnormal that differentiation between sleep and waking by EEG criteria was not possible. The rem percentage in these patients might be spuriously high since many of these patients were taking phenobarbital for seizures chronically, but had had the drug withdrawn 24 to 48 hours prior to recording.

The most detailed study of the sleep patterns of mentally retarded persons to date is that of Feinberg, Braun, and Shulman (1969b). By studying individuals for four or five nights they showed that retarded patients showed a rather marked first night effect, that is, a lower rem percentage on first than on later nights. Feinberg and his co-workers pointed out that the study of Petre-Quadens and Jouvet (1967) only monitored first nights. By restricting analysis to the latter three nights of sleep, Feinberg and his co-workers have provided more meaningful results. All their subjects were adults. Ten mongols were studied; they showed a normal total sleep time for young adults, a moderate decrease in rem percentage, a normal amount of stage 4 time, and a long first nonrem period. Six adults with PKU had a normal total sleep time, a statistically significant decrease in rem percentage, and a long first nonrem period. Patients with MR of unknown etiology had a normal total sleep time, a wide variation in the amount of rem sleep, and the length of the first nonrem period was normal. All these types of MR had a decreased amount of spindle activity and abnormal appearing K-complexes during nonrem stage 2 as compared to normal young adults.

EPILEPSY

In some cases of seizure disorder, epileptic discharges become more frequent as the patient falls asleep. If epilepsy is suspected in a patient whose waking EEG is normal, most clinical electroencephalographers recommend a recording during sleep (Gibbs and Gibbs, 1947; Silverman and Morisaki, 1958). By sleep recording, the clinical electroencephalography does not mean an all-night study. A few minutes of drowsiness and nonrem stages 1 and 2 during a spontaneous or drug induced nap suffices. Nasopharyngeal electrodes which sample the electrical activity of the medial temporal regions of the brain "almost invariably" register seizure discharge during the nonrem sleep of epileptic patients (deJesus and Masland, 1970). A rare patient has epileptiform discharges occurring continuously throughout nonrem sleep (Patry et al., 1971).

All-night recordings reveal that in most epileptic patients, seizure discharges almost disappear during rem sleep (reviewed by Pompeiano, 1969). A marked decrease of epileptiform activity occurs during the rem state of most patients with petit mal (Ross et al., 1966) and with temporal lobe seizures (Kikuchi, 1969). Prolonged telemetric recording during sleep and waking suggests that suppression of epileptiform activity in petit mal patients not only occurs during rem sleep but also occurs episodically every 90 to 120 minutes during waking (Stevens et al., 1971). Though most temporal lobe seizure patients show a depression of seizure discharge during rem periods, rare patients have seizures which begin during a rem period; the seizure aura can be incorporated into the mental activity of the rem state (Epstein and Hill, 1966; Epstein, 1967). In some epileptic patients flashing lights trigger seizure discharges. As the patient falls into nonrem sleep, this photosensitivity falls markedly; results of photic stimulation during rem sleep vary from laboratory to laboratory (see Yamamoto et al., 1971). An experimental seizure disorder can be produced by the intracortical injection of alumina gel. Preliminary studies suggest that the site of this experimental epileptic focus can determine if seizure discharge is more frequent during rem or during nonrem sleep; two monkeys with frontal lobe experimental foci had increased seizure activity during nonrem stages while three monkeys with temporal lobe foci had greater epileptiform spiking during rem sleep (Frank and Pegram, 1970).

Sleep deprivation makes seizures more frequent. This has been used

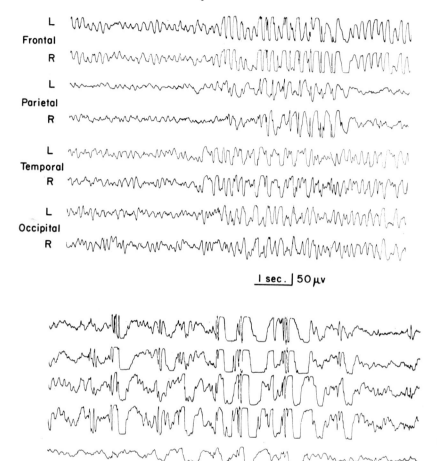

L
Frontal
R

L
Parietal
R

L
Temporal
R

L
Occipital
R

‍I sec. ⌐ 50 μv

Figure 17. Clinical recordings from a patient with petit mal seizures during waking (top tracing) and nonrem sleep. The petit mal discharges become more frequent but shorter in duration in nonrem sleep.

clinically; for example, in a suspected epileptic with normal EEG, sleep deprivation has been employed to bring out the EEG abnormality. Since seizure discharge is more frequent during sleep, one might think that the increased likelihood of sleep during a recording period following sleep deprivation might explain this effect. However, controlled studies indicate this is not the entire explanation (Mattson et al., 1965; Pratt et al., 1967; Geller et al., 1969). Studies in experimental animals from several species indicate that deprivation of the rem type of sleep decreases the threshold to or increases the severity of electrically induced seizures (see Chapter 5).

Preliminary studies have suggested that patients with temporal lobe epilepsy have decreased amounts of slow wave sleep (Greenberg and Pearlman, 1968). Whether this is a function of the patient's worry about the technical apparatus of the sleep laboratory or an inherent sleep disorder, only further studies can determine. An intrinsic sleep disorder is unquestionably present in the degenerative neurologic condition or conditions termed progressive myoclonus epilepsy; sleep is deranged, the nonrem sleep EEG is abnormal, and rem sleep cannot even be detected (Gambi et al., 1970; Hambert and Petersen, 1970).

Two major conclusions emerge from the many studies of sleep and epilepsy: (1) in most seizure patients, epileptiform discharges occur more frequently in nonrem than in rem sleep, and (2) sleep deprivation lowers seizure threshold.

SCHIZOPHRENIA

"Let the dreamer walk about and act like one awakened and we have the clinical picture of dementia praecox," said Carl Gustav Jung, and many before and since him have tried to relate sleep and dreaming to schizophrenia. Bliss, Clark, and West (1959) compared acute schizophrenic psychosis and the symptoms of experimental sleep deprivation; they reported two schizophrenics whose acute psychoses began following severe insomnia. Modern polygraphic studies have confirmed this clinical impression of decreased total sleep time during the early phases of acute schizophrenic psychosis; in addition the sleep which is obtained at this time has a low rem percentage (Snyder, 1969; Kupfer et al., 1970c).

Schizophrenia was one of the first disorders to be studied with the rem/nonrem techniques. Dement (1955) found that reports obtained from rem awakenings in schizophrenic patients had none of the fantasy and drama of normal rem mentation. Most studies of chronic schizophrenia have found the rem percentage to be within normal limits (Caldwell and Domino, 1967; Stern et al., 1969). However, Gulevich et al. (1967) studied thirteen schizophrenic patients who had either recovered from an acute psychosis or were improving and found an increased amount of rem sleep, an average of 116 minutes or 27.4 percent. Nine of the patients had higher rem percentages than the highest rem percentage in a group of seven control subjects. In addition, the first rem period occurred earlier in the night in the schizophrenics, a phenomenon also seen by Stern et al. (1969) in eight acutely ill schizophrenics. Rem percentage is also normal in childhood autistic psychosis, a disorder many clinicians feel may be schizophrenia with onset in childhood (Onheiber et al., 1965; Ornitz et al., 1969; Caldwell et al., 1970).

Schizophrenics do, however, show a decrease in the amount of slow wave sleep, nonrem stages 3 and 4 (Feinberg et al., 1969a; Caldwell, 1969). Caldwell (1969) found that twenty-five schizophrenics of average age thirty-three had a stage 4 percentage of 8 compared to a stage 4 percentage of 15 in ten normal medical students with average age twenty-four. Caldwell was able to divide his patients into fifteen who had a normal amount of stage 4 and ten who had no stage 4 at all, suggesting two types of schizophrenia or two stages in its pathogenesis, at least regarding sleep. Sleep patterns were completely normal in the larger group of patients, while the group with absent stage 4 also had a decreased stage 3 sleep. This lack of slow wave sleep was made up by an increased amount of nonrem stage 2; rem percentage was normal. Unfortunately, Caldwell gave no information that might suggest a clinical differentiation of these two schizophrenic subgroups.

In summary, insomnia and a decreased rem percentage characterizes the early phases of the acute schizophrenic psychosis. The original expectation that rem sleep would show some dramatic abnormality in schizophrenia has not been fulfilled. The hallucinations of delirium tremens may be related to increased amounts of rem sleep; the hallucinations of schizophrenia are not.

DEPRESSION

The term depression refers not only to a disease but to a symptom. Everyone feels blue when things go badly; everyone grieves at the loss of a family member. In addition, though, depression refers to a disease process, probably several specific disease entities. Sometimes the grief reaction can last so long and involve such dissipation of mental energy, such loss of motor activity, and such feelings of worthlessness that it becomes a definite pathological state. More dramatic is the occurrence of depression without significant loss, a depression which seems to come on without apparent cause, sometimes called endogenous depression. Sometimes the guilt feelings can be so much greater than the imagined wrongdoing as to approach psychotic delusions. The differentiation between psychotic and nonpsychotic depression is not always clearcut. A rather clearly outlined subgroup of depressive patients is formed by those individuals who suffer alternating periods of depression and mania. During his manic periods this individual is buoyant, confident, and talkative, progressing to excitement, confusion, and the undertaking of grandiose and unrealistic plans. Manic depressive psychosis is probably inherited (Winokur and Reich, 1970).

The classical clinical descriptions of depression by Hippocrates, Plutarch, and Burdon included a disorder of sleep. The most characteristic sleep problem is early morning awakening; the patient awakes at 0400 or 0500 and cannot return to sleep. Clinical opinion, gleaned from patient reports, suggests that early morning awakening is more characteristic of endogenous than reactive depression (Haider, 1968). Because of the obvious sleep disorder in depression, a number of polygraphic studies have been performed in depressive patients. The early all-night electroencephalographic studies of Diaz-Guerrero and co-workers (1946) and of Zung et al. (1964) utilized the sleep scoring system of Loomis which obscures a clear description of rem sleep; the data of these studies does not contradict the rem/nonrem studies which will be reviewed now.

Hartmann (1968) studied six manic-depressives. Manic periods were associated with decreased total sleep time and rem percentage; depressed periods had a normal total sleep time, an increased rem percentage, and a shortened rem latency. Stage 4 sleep was slightly below normal limits in both manic and depressed states. Gresham and his co-workers (1965) studied the sleep of eight patients admitted to a general referral hospital because of depression. The patients showed greater sleep latency, increased awakenings and time awake, and decreased stage 4 when compared to a control group of age matched hospital employees. Four of these patients were studied again when their depression had improved, and all these measures had returned toward but did not reach normal. The rem percentage of these patients increased from 23.5, 20.6, 24.4, and 18.2 during the height of the depression to 26.7, 28.2, 29.4, and 25.1 respectively during recovery. While each of these values is within normal limits, the direction of change is upward in each case. Mendels and Hawkins (1967) studied twenty-one depressed patients upon admission to the hospital, comparing results to fifteen age-matched control subjects. The patients took longer to fall asleep, woke earlier in the morning, had more time awake and more frequent awakenings, and had a marked decrease in the amount of slow wave sleep. In psychotic depressives, rem percent decreased from the control values of 102 minutes or 23 percent of sleep to 33 minutes or only 8.7 percent of sleep. These authors (1970) have reported a woman who developed a psychotic depression following the death of her father. She had a decreased total sleep time and a total absence of slow wave sleep during the height of depression, but following electroconvulsive treatment and clinical improvement, these values returned to normal. This patient's rem percentage was normal during the depression but rose and was consistently elevated for a number of nights, usually above 30 percent during recovery. Snyder (1969) has reported that psychotic depressives have a decreased rem percentage when entering depression, but an elevated rem percentage and a shortened rem latency during recovery. Snyder suggested that part of the clinical picture of psychotic depression could be related to rem deprivation, with clinical improvement concomitant with a rem "rebound" similar to that seen during recovery from experimental rem deprivation. Vogel and his co-workers (1968) experimentally deprived depressed patients of rem sleep and failed to see any clinical worsening. These polygraphic findings may be related to Miller's (1969) finding that patients during their depression stated that their dreams were happy or of a bland nature, but during recovery their dreams became troubled. Lowry and his co-workers (1971) followed the sleep patterns of six depressed patients for prolonged periods. Five of the six patients had decreased amounts of slow wave sleep while depressed with return to normal levels prior to or concomitant with clinical improvement. Changes in rem sleep in these patients was variable.

In summary, one might conclude that depression entails many types of sleep disorder. Manic-depressives have abnormal sleep characterized by decreased sleeping time and rem percentage during mania and normal sleep time and increased rem during depression. Many but not all patients with severe depression, possibly psychotic depression and possibly exogenous, have early morning awakening and markedly decreased slow wave sleep. Frequently, recovery from depression is accompanied by an increase in rem percentage and a decrease in rem latency.

Chapter 10

THEORIES OF SLEEP

We know that sleep is a state of rest during which the highest centres, subserving consciousness, are functionally separated from the lower centres, motor and sensory. During this state of rest there is a renewal of nutrition, which has been impaired during activity beyond the restorative capacity of the immediate metabolic changes. But rest of the nerve structures is not complete inactivity; this is probably incompatible with any molecular change, even restorative. This renewal entails some activity, without which it could not occur. This gentle function seems to be in ordered form, such as that which constitutes a dream.

SIR WILLIAM GOWERS, 1907

WHY THEORY?

THERE are about as many theories of sleep as there are sleep researchers. For every research worker who has restrained himself from publishing his theoretical ideas on sleep, another investigator has advanced two or more different, often competing, theories. Some sciences, medieval medicine is an example, have been deformed by too early and too extensive theorization. The development of sleep research, however, has reached the point where some type of general theory is desperately needed to hold together such disparate findings. "Never before in the history of biological research," Dement (1966) has said, "has so much been known about something from a descriptive point of view with so little known at the same time about its function." According to the U.C.L.A. Brain Information Service, over six hundred scientific articles are published each year in the field of sleep research. The lack of a comprehensive theoretical framework upon which to hang all these physiologic, pharmacologic, biochemical, psychologic, and clinical observations fragments the field and prevents an overview of sleep phenomenology. The first nine chapters of this book reviewed experimental findings and avoided theory. This final chapter reviews existing sleep theories and adds another.

THEORIES OF SLEEP ORGANIZATION

Most sleep theories can be divided into two types based upon whether they describe the how or the why of sleep. How theories attempt to delineate how we fall asleep, how we move from nonrem to rem sleep, how we awaken. Why theories try to examine the function of one or both of the sleep states. This section will be concerned with how theories, theories of the neural control and organization of sleep.

An earlier era in sleep research saw a controversy between the "active" and "passive" theories of how animals fall asleep. The "active" theory emphasized Hess's observation that electrical stimulation of the medial thalamus can induce sleep; an active, sleep producing neural mechanism was postulated. The "passive" theory held that a decrease in excitatory impulses in the ascending reticular activating system caused sleep; sleep was seen as the absence of wakefulness. While the reticular activating system, as discussed in Chapter 6, plays a major role in awakening, there can be no doubt that sleep induction is a complex phenomenon involving circadian, behavioral, and humoral factors as well as active sleep producing neural circuits. Chapter 3 reviewed some of the studies which have attempted to define the specific brain regions or neurochemical systems responsible for sleep onset, sleep maintenance, and the switch from nonrem to rem sleep. Separate formal theories of sleep organization have been offered by Hernandez-Peon (1965), Koella (1967, 1972), Hartmann (1967, 1969), Torda (1967, 1969), Zanchetti (1969), Jouvet (1969, 1972), Andersson et al. (1971b), and others. The recent Maele symposium on basic sleep mechanisms chaired by Olga Petre-Quadens (1972) analyzed several sleep organization theories in detail. While there is no question that brain stem regions such as the midbrain tegmentum, the pontine raphe nuclei, and the nucleus of the solitary tract play important roles in sleep behavior, the identification of sleep or waking "centers" seems an impossible task. The present reviewer agrees with Koella (1967) when he emphasizes the integration of many brain regions in sleep phenomenology:

> Single functional units do not sleep: they are either active in a particular manner or inactive, and by the very degree, quality, and time pattern of their activity contribute to the whole phenomenon of sleep. Miosis is a typical sleep sign, yet the iris muscles, which through their

specific action bring about the narrowing of the pupil, do not sleep; nor do the pyramidal cells in the motor cortex; but again their discharge pattern is characteristic for sleep. It is the whole organism that sleeps; sleep is an integrative phenomenon. (Koella, 1967, p. 75)

In discussing sleep organization one must note the interesting concept that the rem-nonrem dichotomy of sleep might also extend to wakefulness. The cyclic alteration of brain states which occurs during sleep might continue during wakefulness but might be harder to discern (Kleitman, 1963, 1969; Hartmann, 1968). Some limited evidence for a rem-like state during wakefulness has been uncovered in the study of daytime polygraphic recording (Globus, 1966; Othmer et al., 1969).

Several sleep authorities have detected a shift in emphasis in sleep research. Aserinsky (1967), Dement (1969), and others predict that we cannot understand sleep until we understand the neural mechanism underlying each of the phasic events of sleep: the eye movements, PGO waves, muscular twitches, sleep spindles, K-complexes, phasic EMG depressions, and the momentary changes in mental activity and in spontaneous neuronal discharge rate which sometimes accompany these brief electrical and behavioral events. Grosser and Siegal (1971) suggest that sleep scientists should divide sleep into two types: sleep associated with a phasic event and sleep between two phasic events. The rem and nonrem division of sleep, they conclude, is obsolete.

FUNCTIONS OF SLEEP

Before considering possible functions of sleep one must ask if sleep has a function. Are we studying an interesting but functionless phenomenon? Could we do away with sleep altogether? In a discussion of circadian rest-activity rhythms, Aschoff (1965) pointed out how animals adapted to temporal as well as geographic ecological niches. Some animals are adapted to nocturnal existence while others, like man, to a diurnal one. Many species hunt in the daytime but are essentially helpless in the dark against nocturnal predators. A system of reversible coma might evolve to keep diurnal animals in their hiding places during the hours of darkness. Some workers have suggested that sleep in modern man is an evolutionary throwback, a physiologic appendix; modern man could stay awake all the time, work all day, play all night. If common sense does not counteract any such suggestion, a review of the sleep deprivation studies discussed in Chapter 5 will. In one sense, then, the function of sleep is to prevent the occurrence of sleep deprivation symptoms. One would prefer a more detailed exposition of sleep's function. There have been two basic approaches to this refinment of sleep's function, one biochemical and one psychologic.

Some have suggested that some nervous molecular species is used during wakefulness at a rate faster than it can be replenished. During sleep the reverse occurs. This has been facetiously termed the "bottle" theory. As the day progresses the level of this unknown substance falls, as if its level was falling in a container. When the person sleeps, the level rises. Sleep beyond a certain amount, the full bottle, is no longer therapeutic. Sleep deprivation causes the level to drop to a danger point and symptomatology occurs. The "filling of the bottle" is presumed to be an energy-requiring process since brain oxygen consumption does not decrease as one falls asleep. Chapter 5 reviewed the biochemical studies attempting to discover the contents of the bottle. Whole brain content of high energy phosphate compounds is higher in sleeping than in sleep-deprived animals. The marked drowsiness which occurs following a seizure may possibly be related to these observations since experimental seizures in animals are associated with a marked fall in brain high energy phosphate levels, an emptying of the bottle. The incorporation of phosphate into phosphoprotein and phosphopeptides is also increased in brain but not other organs during sleep. Others have suggested that neurotransmitter substances are used more rapidly during wakefulness, and their stores are replenished during sleep. The neurochemical approach has been criticized most thoroughly by Kleitman (1963), who felt that the grogginess many people feel after arising was not compatible with the "full bottle." From the still fragmentary initial efforts in this area, many chemical changes occur in the nervous system during sleep, and some of these may be related to sleep's function or functions.

Throughout history, from the cult of Aesculapius to the cult of Freud, people have considered sleep to have a psychologic function or functions. Sleep provides a time when events of the preceding day can be repeated and rehearsed without extraneous intervening environmental occurrences. This information processing sorts the day residue, discarding that which does not fit with previous formulations or prejudices, and arranging properly that which correlates with material already on file. One of Freud's key observations was that each period of sleep mentation contains elements of events from the preceding day and elements of events from many years before, particularly from childhood. Attempts to describe the psychologic functions of sleep have been carried out almost entirely in man, of course, while chemical studies have been performed in experimental animals. The functions of sleep may incorporate both these approaches either independent of or isomorphic to one another. Mandell and Spooner (1968) recommended the comparison of biochemical changes in animal brains with psychologic changes in man during normal and altered sleep as one of the basic psychochemical research strategies to discover chemical events underlying thought processes.

Many theoreticians have assumed that the rest or renewal theories previously applied to sleep in general now apply to nonrem sleep alone. Hobson (1969) argues that the increase in slow wave sleep which occurs following exercise "substantiates the commonsense rest theory of sleep." Concomitantly, a great many papers have totally ignored any possible function of nonrem sleep (probably assuming that nonrem has something to do with "rest" or neurochemical renewal) and have advanced theories for the function of rem sleep. Roffwarg, Muzio, and Dement (1966) suggest that the rem state is important in the normal development of sensory portions of the brain *in utero* and in neonatal life. They postulate that "the rem mechanism serves as an endogenous source of stimulation, furnishing great quantities of functional excitation to higher centers" which "assist in structural maturation and differentiation of key sensory and motor areas within the central nervous system." While this ingenious hypothesis may explain the high levels of rem sleep seen in the neonate, it cannot be the sole function of the rem state. This complex state in the adult must be more than a physiologic umbilical scar, a reminder of intra-uterine life.

Biologically oriented psychoanalysts have attempted to adapt psychoanalytic dream theory to polygraphic sleep studies (Altshuler, 1966; Jones, 1970). While many have merely equated freudian dream psychology with rem sleep, other psychoanalysts have pointed out that the mental experiences of nonrem sleep cannot be ignored by any inclusive theory of sleep and dreaming (see, for example, Trosman, 1963). The symposium chaired by Kramer (1969) presented separate attempts to consolidate polygraphic findings with several different schools (Jungian, Adlerian, focal conflict, culturalist, existentialist) of psychoanalytic dream psychology. Several separate theories have related rem sleep to memory. Dewan (1969, 1970) postulated that the rem state "represents the physiological concomitant of a spontaneous self-programming process in the brain." Greenberg (1970) theorized that the rem state "serves to transfer recent perceptions from the perceptual areas, or short-term memory stores, to areas for long-term memory storage, clearing the perceptual areas so that they would be free for new perceptions." Rem sleep is a time when events of the day are played back from a real-time tape recorded to a much slower recorder, he proposes; this memory transfer prevents the perceptual areas from any ongoing environmental interaction. Pearlman (1970) takes this one step further when he suggests that the rem state is the time when intellectual insight becomes emotional insight. By studying mental content of several rem periods of the same night, Kramer and his co-workers (1964) have developed the concept that successive rem periods provide "tension accumulation, discharge, and regression." Physiologists have emphasized that no psychoanalytic formulation can explain the extent of the rem state through ontogeny and phylogeny. Are neonates and opossums expressing unconscious wishes during their rem periods?

Other workers have tried to compare sleep's dichotomy to other dichotomies. Iskander and Kaebling (1970) compared nonrem and rem states to the trophotrophic and ergotrophic states of Hess and Gellhorn. West (1969) suggested that nonrem sleep is a catabolic state which dissipates metabolic products accumulated during waking, while rem sleep is an anabolic state which replaces substrates depleted during wakefulness. Rechtschaffen et al. (1963) have compared rem mentation to the primary process thinking and nonrem mentation to the secondary process thinking of psychoanalytic theory. Schapiro (1967) suggested a theory of differential data processing, symbolic processing during the rem state, and cognitive processing during the nonrem state. Gaarder (1966) pointed out that two types of information are stored in a computer, data and instructions which tell what operations to perform on the data. The human computer puts data into storage during nonrem sleep, he suggests, but during rem, instructions to the self are processed, changing a person's character.

Could rem sleep be some sort of response to nonrem sleep? Several separate theories have developed from the general hypothesis that prolonged nonrem sleep could be harmful to the sleeping organism unless periodically punctuated by the rem state. Ephron and Carrington (1966) suggested that prolonged inactivity of the neocortex was detrimental and that rem sleep represented a homeostatic mechanism to increase "cortical tonus" without awakening. Berger (1969) proposed that "rem sleep provides a mechanism for the establishment of neuromuscular pathways in voluntary conjugate eye movements." Ullman (1958) and Snyder (1966) postulated that animals sleeping in the wild had to awaken frequently to survey their environment for the presence of predators and that rem sleep might provide preparatory activation of the nervous system prior to each awakening. All these theories are compatible with the idea that the function of sleep, if any, occurs during the nonrem state and that each rem period could be replaced by a period of wakefulness (with waking eye movements according to Berger). Many studies have been performed over the years, as summarized in Chapter 5, in which sleepers were awakened whenever they entered a rem period; when these subjects are then allowed to repose undisturbed, their rem sleep is not unchanged or even decreased, as these theories predict, but it increases over baseline levels. Studies in the rat (Webb and Friedmann, 1971) and cat (Ursin, 1968) relate the duration of each rem period to the duration of the previous nonrem period or a substage of it and have been interpreted as supporting theories such as those proposed by Ephron and Carrington (1966) and Berger (1969). This relationship does not hold in primates, however. The first nightly rem period in man is the shortest, yet it always follows the longest period of nonrem sleep. As discussed in Chapter 4, the first rem period of the all-night sleep of the chimpanzee is shorter than the last rem period, yet it usually follows several hours of nonrem sleep including most or all of the nightly accumulations of slow wave sleep. Whitehead and his coworkers (1969) found the same rem percentage during night sleep after a day of quiet wakefulness and after a day filled with naps of nonrem sleep. In addition, there may be some species such as the spiny anteater who have much nonrem sleep and no rem sleep at all.

In my opinion, available evidence favors discarding any functional sleep theories which postulate that rem sleep arises as a reaction or adaption to nonrem sleep.

Despite the loss of these few theories, many biochemical, psychologic, computer processing theories remain. I would like to now present my own hypothesis to explain why there are two types of sleep (Freemon, 1970) and then return to put all these remaining separate theories in perspective.

RECIPROCAL ENVIRONMENTAL SURVEILLANCE MODEL

I suggest that there are two types of sleep because there are two separate arousal systems. One system surveys the environment during nonrem sleep and "rests" during rem; the other system, the larger, "rests" during nonrem sleep and assumes environmental surveillance during the rem state. The details of the term "rest" are yet to be determined, part neurochemical, part data processing, but the main postulated characteristic of this hypothetical renewal process is that neural tissue undergoing rest and rejuvenation cannot participate in environmental surveillance.

The theory accepts and expands on two previous formulations. Wilson and Zung (1966) have argued that vigilance, that is, the ability to record and process environmental information for signals of impending danger, decreases during sleep but never reaches zero. They postulate two systems of vigilance, the normal one present during waking and a much smaller one, perhaps contained within the larger, which is active throughout sleep. Routtenberg (1966, 1968) has reviewed the evidence that the brain may contain two separate arousal systems. His arousal system I is the classical arousal system of Moruzzi and Magoun, the ascending reticular activating system. His arousal system II, developed from the anatomical studies of Nauta (1958) and the stimulation-reward system of Olds (1962), consists of limbic structures including septal nuclei, median forebrain bundle, and hippocampus. He postulates that these two hypothetical systems are mutually inhibitory, and both are required for memory.

All theories of sleep emphasize certain areas of data and deemphasize (disregard?) other areas. The reciprocal environmental surveillance model of sleep is based upon these two sets of experimental findings:

1. Certain brain regions show slow electrical activity during nonrem sleep and fast during rem while others show the opposite or reciprocal pattern, fast activity during nonrem, slow during rem sleep. A general rule in electroencephalography holds that slow electrical activity in a brain area usually indicates relative inactivity of that region. The classic example of this phenomenon is the replacement of slow by fast activity in neocortex accompanied by a change from sleeping to waking following electrical stimulation of the reticular formation (Moruzzi and Magoun, 1949). Hippocampal theta in the cat, rabbit, and other animals during waking may be an exception to this rule, though the present formulation agrees with Rhodes (1969), Bennett (1971), and other authorities that the appearance of this rhythm represents an inhibited hippocampus.

2. During sleep, both types of sleep, man surveys the environment and can awaken on preset cues. Most formulations of sleep have emphasized how much the sleeping man or animal has withdrawn from his environment; he is said to be unconscious, deafferented, attending to internal cues. I would like to emphasize the surprising ability of the sleeper to analyze environmental events and act on them. Sleep is not coma. The loss of memory which sometimes accompanies these responses makes the introspective thinker deemphasize environmental interaction. Yet, as reviewed in Chapter 6, considerable scientific data has validated the ability of the sleeper to process environmental information, at least to the extent that danger signals will awaken.

Now the reciprocal environmental surveillance model of sleep can be stated in detail. Let us define two brain subsystems, whose anatomical components we will identify later. For ease in explanation let us call these systems X and Y. This model assumes a reciprocity of environmental survey function between these two theoretical systems; that is, X samples the environment for danger signals during nonrem sleep periods and Y performs this function during rem sleep periods. While one of these systems analyzes the available stimuli reaching the brain from peripheral sense organs, the other undergoes the presumed process of renewal. This model supposes that the renewal process, whatever its biochemical or physiologic nature, eliminates the tissue undergoing the process from participating in the reception and analysis of ongoing information. The model states that during rem periods, X undergoes renewal while Y surveys incoming data; these two systems then reciprocate function during nonrem periods. Take the example of the new mother who sleeps undisturbed by the familiar roar and whistle of the passing train but who awakens to her baby's soft crying. In rem periods, when the train passes, Y analyzes this sound and dismisses it, but when it encounters the baby's cry, Y activates X from its renewal process and the brain awakes.

One may analogize this mechanism to a "military model" in which the brain contains two "sentries." One sentry stands guard while the other sleeps like a log beside him, exhausted from the day's military maneuvers. After a specified period, the sentry, Private X, gently nudges the sleeper, Private Y, who then assumes the surveillance duties while X retires. This reciprocating rest and sentry duty continues throughout the night unless one of the sentries, say Y, becomes suspicious of an environmental occurrence, be it sight, sound, or smell, that might indicate danger. In this case, Y awakens the sleeping X and the rest of the camp to further investigate this disturbance. Should the disturbance prove ephemeral, the camp settles down again, and after a time Y resumes his lonely sentry post; or perhaps if the disturbance occurred near the end of the prescribed duty period, Y retires and X begins his turn on guard.

Lack of knowledge of the renewal process hampers the anatomical delineation of these surveillance systems. Eventually a chemical description of the renewal process may be possible, though this phenomenon could be more associated with some type of information filing and less with chemical changes. At our present state of knowledge, unit activity rates fail to identify the renewal process. Spike bursts could indicate increased activity, or they could represent loss of inhibition because inhibitory neurons are undergoing renewal, as suggested by Eccles (1961). The renewal or regenerative function could be related to glial metabolism as shown by Hyden and Lange (1963) and could be unaffected by neuronal firing rates. Certainly if we can establish the relationship of unit activity to renewal, we will have a powerful tool to identify the two sentry systems since neurons of these systems may mingle in the same anatomic location or nucleus. At the present time we must rely on gross electrophysiologic recording to identify the reciprocating arousal systems.

During nonrem sleep most brain regions show slow waves. These areas include neocortex, most of the reticular core, many thalamic nuclei, basal ganglia, and in man most of the hippocampus and hippocampal complex. This slow activity is presumed to represent the renewal process. These same areas show fast activity during rem sleep and may at that time be registering and analyzing environmental events for danger signals. These brain regions are then part of system Y, undergoing renewal during nonrem sleep and standing guard duty during rem. Note that system Y contains some limbic areas. The neocortex shows some slow activity in the theta frequency band during the rem state. It is likely, then, that some cellular components of neocortex are in system Y, and some are in system X.

Certain regions show slow activity, usually in the theta range, during rem sleep. These regions in man, reviewed in Chapter 4, include posterior hypothalamus, certain thalamic nuclei, and limited and variable portions of the anterior hippocampus. These same regions show fast activity in nonrem sleep. This formulation suggests that these brain regions form system X, undergoing renewal during rem sleep and serving as sentry during nonrem. Studies in carnivores and rodents reviewed in Chapter 3 suggest that other portions of this system may be septal nuclei, periacqueductal gray matter, limbic midbrain area of Nauta, and caudal brain stem. Future depth electrode studies in man and animals may aid in further anatomic delineation of these two systems.

Nonhuman primates do not have this reciprocal environmental surveillance system. The phenomenon most characteristic of the sleep of nonhuman primates is the protected sleeping environment. Even chimpanzees who forage widely in grasslands during the day return to the forests to sleep in trees at night. Man, even the most primitive men living today, do not sleep in trees. Perhaps the dual arousal system was lost early in primate evolution, restricting primates to protected sleeping sites to escape prowling nocturnal carnivores. I propose that early protohominoids were tree sleeping primates. The deforestation which accompanied successive ice ages forced protoman down from the trees. His poorly developed dual arousal system caused him to be easy prey to hunting beasts at night. Only a very few survived each ice age, only the very smartest, the best organized. With reforestation in each interglacial age protoman became more plentiful. Finally, modern man, emerging after the last ice age, had redeveloped the basic mammalian pattern of the dual environmental surveillance sleep system. In terms of his sleep, man has many basic primate attributes and some characteristics of carnivores and other nonprimate mammals.

The present framework absorbs many previous sleep models. The biochemical and physiologic theories of sleep renewal, which the recognition of sleep's duality relegated from total sleep time to nonrem sleep periods, the present formulation redistributes to a theoretical system X during rem and a system Y during nonrem. Berger's idea that rem sleep provides exercise for the eye muscles might have an element of truth; in addition, one notes that the neck muscles relax completely during rem but are active in nonrem in many species including man. Neck and eye muscle relaxation and activity parallel the reciprocity of brain systems X and Y. The environmental surveillance model, restricted to adult animals, can incorporate the ontogenetic theory of Roffwarg and co-workers (1966), which limits itself to fetal and neonatal life. Often ontogenesis adapts for developmental use structures which have important adult functions. Workers who study the neuroanatomic substrate and neurochemical mechanisms by which a sleeping individual progresses from nonrem to rem periods or vice versa are actually examining the complex mechanism by which one environmental survey system switches to the other. In terms of the "army analogue," these workers are observing "the changing of the guard," certainly an important and often a colorful event. The present framework can also incorporate theories and data concerning the sleep-dream cycle, which suggests that rem and nonrem periods occupy specific times throughout the night and perhaps also throughout the daytime hours. According to the model, workers studying the rem-nonrem cycle are trying to read "the duty roster posted on the guard house door" which tells each sentry when he is on duty. The "two sentries" theory can absorb most aspects of models of differential data processing between the two stages if one assumes that the mentation sampled by dream reports parallels the ongoing internal activity of each surveillance system. Adapting psychoanalytic dream theory to the many phylogenetic and ontogenetic observations on rem sleep has proved difficult. The present model can incorporate psychoanalytic dream theory if one believes that the ongoing mentation of the rem sentry contains material of psychologic import and if one assumes that in late primate evolution the rem environmental survey system

developed internal autistic aspects which give the rem state a psychologic function quite apart from strict environmental surveillance.

This reciprocal environmental surveillance model of sleep can or-
ganize existing data and predict future results in many of the neurologic sciences concerned with sleep research. In the field of neuro-
chemistry, the model predicts that if chemical changes occur in brain
as a result of sleep they will have a regional basis reciprocating between rem and nonrem periods. During recovery from rem deprivation, glycogen decreases in hippocampus and caudal brain stem but
not neocortex (Karadzic and Mrsulja, 1969). The model interprets
these results to show that system X (hippocampus) but not system Y
(neocortex) suffered from inability to undergo the renewal process
during rem deprivation; during recovery, the regenerative process required increased energy expenditure, and glycogen stores decreased.
When neurochemical studies are repeated with regional measurements
and with analysis of sleep stages, the many chemical changes reviewed
in Chapter 5 may show increases in some brain regions during rem
and others during nonrem periods.

In man and the chimpanzee, slow activity predominates in neocortex during the first few nonrem periods while later periods show
mainly K-complexes and spindles. In the human case with posterior
hypothalamic recording discussed in Chapter 4, the slow activity
present in this structure in early rem periods disappeared from later
rem sleep. Studies in man have shown that later rem periods are
longer, have greater eye movements, have greater variations in pulse
and blood pressure, and are associated with more vivid dreaming.
These observations predict that early rem periods and early nonrem
periods are more associated with neurochemical renewal; later sleep
periods are more associated with psychologic changes.

In the field of arousal research, the present model notes that either
unfamiliar signals or signals of known importance awaken much more
rapidly than higher intensity habituated stimuli. The formulation predicts that the type of arousal stimulus which awakens most rapidly
from one type of sleep should not necessarily be the stimulus which
best awakens from the other type of sleep. One might predict that in
primitive macrosomatic animals, olfactory stimuli should awaken more
readily during nonrem sleep and auditory or tactile stimuli should
arouse more quickly during rem sleep. The dual arousal theory pro-

vides a framework for the many findings of the changes in synaptic "transmission" along sensory pathways discussed in Chapter 6.

In the field of sleep mentation analysis, the model suggests that ongoing mental activity during sleep corresponds to the mental activity of the sentry. Dream reports from awakenings from rem periods should enable us to define the mental processes of system Y, the rem sentry. When we can define the anatomic limits of system Y in man we can attribute to this brain subsystem specific thought processes. Similarly, by using mentation reports from awakenings from nonrem periods, particularly periods early in the night in which slow activity predominates, we can analyze the ongoing mentation of isolated brain system X, the nonrem sentry. Psychological studies in waking individuals who are undergoing either rem deprivation or deprivation of nonrem stages 3 and 4 should complement the sleep mentation reports in attributing types of mental activity to specific brain subsystems. For example, rem deprivation should produce reversible dysfunction localized to system X, which undergoes renewal during rem. If the present model proves correct, further sleep research should produce anatomic and psychologic dissection of two subsystems of mentation, separate during sleep but cooperating during wakefulness. Man's forced descent from the trees speeded the evolution of these two neurologic systems underlying two types of mental activity. Perhaps in some people, or in all people at some times, these two systems do not properly cooperate during wakefulness, producing the basic schizoid human predicament described by Koestler (1967).

Actually, of course, the real situation is undoubtedly more complex than this simplified model. We already know that the two sentries do not remain pure throughout the night but change in character, possibly because small portions of one system fulfill their renewal function and can join the other system in environmental surveillance. Nevertheless, the model can absorb as allies most previous formulations of sleep function. The model negates polemics over dreaming during nonrem periods and over the deepest stage of sleep by emphasizing the inherent differences of the mental activity and arousal mechanisms in each sleep stage. The model synthesizes and categorizes previous findings and makes specific predictions in each of the neurologic sciences concerned with sleep research.

SUMMARY

This short monograph has attempted to review the sprawling, diffuse, fascinating, exasperating field of sleep research. Some areas, autonomic physiology is an example, have not been covered in the detail they deserve, but references to the original literature have been provided. For those readers who have plowed through the entire book, I say thank you and welcome to the end. Despite all these pages and words, all this scientific study, we cannot ascribe any function unequivocally to sleep. We all do it every day, but we don't know why. I must agree with Hartmann (1967, p. 144) that such a complex phenomenon as sleep probably has many functions, some neurochemical, some psychologic, some ontogenetic. I have suggested an explanation as to why there might be two kinds of sleep and why human sleep, like many human attributes, seems to be a cross between the sleep of other primates and of carnivores. Why don't you mull over the data and the theories in this book and see if you can come up with a better idea? Sleep on it.

BIBLIOGRAPHY

Adey, WR, FR Bell, and BJ Dennis (1962): Effects of LSD-25, psilocybin, and psilocin on temporal lobe EEG patterns and learned behavior in the cat. *Neurol, 12:*591-602.

Adey, WR, E Bors, and RW Porter (1968): EEG sleep patterns after high cervical lesions in man. *Arch Neurol, 19:*377-383.

Adey, WR, CW Dunlop, and CE Hendrix (1960): Hippocampal slow waves: Distribution and phase relationships in the course of approach learning. *Arch Neurol, 3:*74-90.

Adey, WR, RT Kado, and JM Rhodes (1963): Sleep: Cortical and subcortical recordings in the chimpanzee. *Science, 141:*932-933.

Adey, WR, DO Walter, and CE Hendrix (1961): Computer techniques in correlation and spectral analyses of cerebral slow waves during discriminative behavior. *Exp Neurol, 3:*501-524.

Adey, WR, DO Walter, and DF Lindsley (1962): Subthalamic lesions: Effect on learned behavior and correlated hippocampal and subcortical slow-wave activity. *Arch Neurol, 6:*194-207.

Agnew, HW Jr, and WB Webb (1968a): Sleep patterns of 30 to 39 year old male subjects (abstract). *Psychophysiol, 5:*228.

Agnew, HW Jr, and WB Webb (1968b): Sleep patterns of the healthy elderly (abstract). *Psychophysiol, 5:*229.

Agnew, HW Jr, WB Webb, and RL Williams (1966): The first night effect: an EEG study of sleep. *Psychophysiol, 2:*263-266.

Agnew, HW Jr, WB Webb, and RL Williams (1967): Sleep patterns in late middle age males: an EEG study. *Electroenceph Clin Neurophysiol, 23:* 168-171

Agnew, HW Jr, WB Webb, and RL Williams (1967): Comparison of stage four and 1-REM sleep deprivation. *Percept Motor Skills, 24:*851-858.

Akindele, MO, JI Evans, and I Oswald (1970): Mono-amine oxidase inhibitors, sleep and mood. *Electroenceph Clin Neurophysiol, 29:*47-56.

Albert, I, GA Cicala, and J Siegel (1970): The behavioral effects of REM sleep deprivation in rats. *Psychophysiol, 6:*550-560.

Allison, T (1965): Cortical and subcortical evoked responses to central stimuli during wakefulness and sleep. *Electroenceph Clin Neurophysiol, 18:*131-139.

Allison, T, WR Goff, and MB Sterman (1966): Cerebral somatosensory responses evoked during sleep in the cat. *Electroenceph Clin Neurophysiol, 21:*461-468.

Altshuler, KZ (1966): Comments on recent sleep research related to psychoanalytic theory. *Arch Gen Psychiat, 15:*235-239.

Amadeo, M, and E Gomez (1966): Eye movements, attention and dreaming in subjects with lifelong blindness. *Canad Psychiat Assoc J, 11*:500-507.

Ambler, E (1938): *Epitaph for a Spy.* London, Hodder and Stoughton (New York, Knopf, 1952).

Andersen, P (1972): Physiological basis of spindle waves. In Olga Petre-Quadens (editor): *Basic Sleep Mechanisms,* in press.

Andersson, SA, E Holmgren, and JR Mason (1917a): Synchronization and desynchronization in the thalamus of the unanesthetized decorticate cat. *Electroenceph Clin Neurophysiol, 31*:335-345.

Andersson, SA, E Holmgren, and JR Mason (1971b): Localized thalamic rhythmicity induced by spinal and cortical lesions. *Electroenceph Clin Neurophysiol, 31*:347-356.

Angeleri, F, GF Marchesi, and A Quattrini (1969): Effects of chronic thalamic lesions on the electrical activity of the neocortex and on sleep. *Arch Ital Biol, 107*:633-667.

Appenzeller, O, and AP Fischer, Jr (1968): Disturbances of rapid eye movements during sleep in patients with lesions of the nervous system. *Electroenceph Clin Neurophysiol, 25*:29-32.

Arduini, A, G Berlucchi, and P Strata, (1963): Pyramidal activity during sleep and wakefulness. *Arch Ital Biol, 101*:530-544.

Arkin, AM, MF Toth, J Baker, and JM Hastey (1970): The frequency of sleep talking in the laboratory among chronic sleep talkers and good dream recallers. *J Nerv Ment Dis, 151*:369-374.

Arkin, AM, ED Weitzman, and JM Hastey (1966): An observational note on eye movement patterns during REM and nonREM sleep in subjects with congenital nystagmus. *Psychophysiol, 3*:69-72.

Armstrong, RH, D Burnap, A Jacobson, A Kales, S Ward, and J Golden (1965): Dreams and gastric secretions in duodenal ulcer patients. *New Physician, 14*:241-243.

Aserinsky, E, and N Kleitman (1955): Two types of ocular motility occurring in sleep. *J Appl Physiol, 8*:1-10.

Aserinsky, E (1967): Physiological activity associated with segments of the rapid eye movement period. In SS Kety, EV Evarts, and HL Williams (editors): *Sleep and Altered States of Consciousness.* Baltimore, Williams and Wilkins, pp. 338-350.

Aschoff, J (1965): Circadian rhythms in man. *Science, 148*:1427-1432.

Baekeland, F (1966): The effect of methyl phenidate on the sleep cycle in man. *Psychopharmacol, 10*:179-183.

Baekeland, F (1967): Pentobarbital and dextroamphetamine sulfate; effects on the sleep cycle in man. *Psychopharmacol, 11*:388-396.

Baekeland, F (1970): Exercise deprivation: sleep and psychological reactions. *Arch Gen Psychiat, 22*:365-369.

Baekeland, F, and R Lasky (1968): The morning recall of rapid eye movement period reports given earlier in the night. *J Nerv Ment Dis, 147:* 570-579.

Baekeland, F, and L Lundwall (1971): Effects of methyldopa on sleep patterns in man. *Electroenceph Clin Neurophysiol, 31*:269-273.

Baekeland, F, R Resch, and D Katz (1968): Presleep mentation and dream reports II: cognitive style, contiguity to sleep, and time of night. *Arch Gen Psychiat, 19*:300-311.

Bakin, H (1970): Sleep walking in twins. *Lancet, 2*:446-447.

Balzano, E, and M Jeannerod (1970): Activite multi-unitaire de structures sous-corticales pendant le cycle veille-sommeil chez le chat. *Electroenceph Clin Neurophysiol, 28*:136-145.

Bancaud, J, J Talarach, M Bordas-Ferrer, JL Auber, and M Marchand (1964): Les acces epileptiques au course du sommeil de nuit (etude stereo-electroencephalographique). *Rev Neurol, 110*:314.

Baust, W, editor (1970): *Ermudung, Schlaff und Traum.* Stuttgart, Wissenschlaftliche Verlagsgesellschaft.

Baust, W, and G Berlucchi (1964): Reflex response to clicks of cat's tensor tympani during sleep and wakefulness and the influence thereon of the auditory cortex. *Arch Ital Biol, 102*:686-712.

Baust, W, G Berlucchi, and G Moruzzi (1964): Changes in the auditory input in wakefulness and during the synchronized and desynchronized stages of sleep. *Arch Ital Biol, 102*:657-674.

Belugou, JL, and O Benoir (1966): Activite unitaire spontanee des noyaux de relais somesthesiques pendant la veille et le sommeil (abstract). *J Physiol (Paris), 58*:461

Bennett, TL (1971): Hippocampal theta activity and behavior: a review. *Comm Behav Biol, 6*:37-48.

Benoir, O (1964): Activite unitaire du nerf optique, du corps genouille lateral et de la formation reticulaire durant les differents stades de sommeil. *J Physiol (Paris), 56*:259-262.

Benoir, O, J Thomas, and JL Belugou (1965): Activite unitaire dans le systeme somesthesique lors de la veille et du sommeil (abstract). *J Physiol (Paris), 57*:223.

Benoit, O (1967): Influences toniques et phasiques exercees par le sommeil sur l'activite de la voie visuelle. *J Physiol (Paris), 59*:295-317.

Bergamasco, B, L Bergamini, T Doriguzzi, and D Fabiani (1968): EEG sleep patterns as a prognostic criterion in post traumatic coma. *Electroenceph Clin Neurophysiol, 24*:374-377.

Berger, FM (1967): Drugs and suicide in the United States. *Clin Pharmacol Therap, 8*:219-223.

Berger, RJ (1961): Tonus of extrinsic laryngeal muscles during sleep and dreaming. *Science, 134*:840.

Berger, RJ (1963): Experimental modification of dream content by meaningful verbal stimuli. *Brit J Psychiat, 109*:722-740.

Berger, RJ (1967): When is a dream is a dream is a dream? *Exp Neurol Suppl, 4*:15-28.

Berger, RJ (1969): Oculomotor control: a possible function of REM sleep. *Psychol Rev, 76*:144-164.

Berger, RJ, and GW Meier (1966): The effects of selective deprivation of states of sleep in the developing monkey. *Psychophysiol, 2*:354-371.

Berger, RJ, P Olley, and I Oswald (1962): The EEG, eye-movements and dreams of the blind. *Quart J Exp Psychol, 14*:183-186.

Berger, RJ, and I Oswald (1962a): Effects of sleep deprivation on behavior, subsequent sleep, and dreaming. *J Mental Sci, 108*:457-465.

Berger, RJ, and I Oswald (1962b): Eye movements during active and passive dreams. *Science, 137*:601.

Berger, RJ, JM Walker, and TD Scott (1970): Characteristics of sleep in the burrowing owl and the tree shrew (abstract). *Psychophysiol, 7*:303.

Berlucchi, G (1965): Callosal activity in unrestrained, unanesthetized cats. *Arch Ital. Biol, 103*:623-634.

Berlucchi, G, G Moruzzi, G Zalvi, and P Strata (1964): Pupil behavior and ocular movements during synchronized and desynchronized sleep. *Arch Ital Biol, 102*:230-244.

Berlucchi, G, JB Munson, and G Rizzolatti (1967): Changes in click-evoked responses in the auditory system and the cerebellum of free-moving cats during sleep and waking. *Arch Ital Biol, 105*:118-135.

Bert, J, H Ayats, A Martino, and H Collomb (1967a): Le sommeil nocturne chez le babouin *Papio papio. Folia primatol, 6*:28-43.

Bert, J, and H Collomb (1966): L'electroencephalogramme du sommeil nocturne chez la babouin: Etude par telemetrie. *J Physiol (Paris), 58*:285-301.

Bert, J, H Collomb, and A Martino (1967b): L'electroencephalogramme de sommeil d'un pro-simien. *Electroenceph Clin Neurophysiol, 23*:342-450.

Bert, J, DF Kripke, and JM Rhodes (1970): Electroencephalogram of the mature chimpanzee: 24-hour recordings. *Electroenceph Clin Neurophysiol, 28*:368-373.

Bertini, M, (1970): *Psicofisiologia del Sonna e del Sogno.* Milan, Editrice Vita e Pensiero.

Bizzi, E (1966): Discharge patterns of single geniculate neurons during the rapid eye movements of sleep. *J Neurophysiol, 29*:1087-1095.

Bizzi, E (1966): Changes in the orthodromic and antidromic response of optic tract during the eye movements of sleep. *J Neurophysiol, 29*:861-870.

Bizzi, E, and DC Brooks (1963): Functional connections between pontine reticular formation and lateral geniculate nucleus during deep sleep. *Arch Ital Biol, 101*:666-680.

Bizzi, E, O Pompeiano, and I Somogyi (1964): Spontaneous activity of single vestibular neurons of unrestrained cats during sleep and wakefulness. *Arch Ital Biol, 102*:308-330.

Bliss, EL, LD Clark, and CD West (1959): Studies of sleep deprivation: relationship to schizophrenia. *Arch Neurol Psychiat, 81*:348-359.

Bogacz, J, and E Wilson (1969): Visual evoked potentials at hypothalamic and tegmental areas of the upper brain stem. *Electroenceph Clin Neurophysiol, 26:*288-295.

Bowers, MB Jr, EL Hartmann, and DX Freedman (1966): Sleep deprivation and brain acetyl choline. *Science, 153:*1416-1417.

Boyaner, HG (1970): Effects of REM sleep deprivation on exploration in rats. *Psychol Rep, 27:*918.

Brannen, JO, and RE Jewett (1969): Effects of selected phenothiazines on REM sleep in schizophrenics. *Arch Gen Psychiat, 21:*284-290.

Brazier, MAB (1967): Absence of dreaming or failure to recall? *Exp Neurol Suppl, 4:*91-98.

Brazier, MAB (1968): Studies of the EEG activity of limbic structures in man. *Electroenceph Clin Neurophysiol, 25:*309-318.

Brebbia, DR, KZ Altschuler, and NS Kline (1969): Lithium and the electroencephalogram during sleep. *Dis Nerv Syst, 30:*541-546.

Bremer, F (1935): "Cerveau isole" et physiologie du sommeil. *Compt Rend Soc Biol, 118:*1235-1241.

Bricolo, A, G Turella, CA Mazza, P Buffatti, and JC Grosslercher (1970): Modificazioni del sonno notturno in parkinsoniani trattati con L-dopa. *Sistema Nervoso, 22:*181-190.

Brodal, A (1969): *Neurological Anatomy: Its Relation to Clinical Medicine.* New York, Oxford University Press.

Brooks, DC (1967): Localization of the lateral geniculate nucleus monophasic waves associated with paradoxical sleep in the cat. *Electroenceph Clin Neurophysiol, 23:*123-133.

Brooks, DC (1968): Waves associated with eye movement in the awake and sleeping cat. *Electroenceph Clin Neurophysiol, 24:*532-541.

Brooks, DC, and E Bizzi (1963): Brain stem electrical activity during deep sleep. *Arch Ital Biol, 101:*648-665.

Brooks, DC and MD Gershon (1971): Eye movement potentials in the oculomotor and visual systems of the cat: a comparison of reserpine induced waves with those present during wakefulness and rapid eye movement sleep. *Brain Res, 27:*223-239.

Broughton, RJ (1968): Sleep disorders: disorders of arousal? *Science, 159:*1070-1078.

Broughton, RJ, R Poire, and CA Tassinari (1965): The electrodermogram (Tarchanoff effect) during sleep. *Electroenceph Clin Neurophysiol, 18:*691-708.

Brown, BB (1968): Frequency and phase of hippocampal theta activity in the spontaneously behaving cat. *Electroenceph Clin Neurophysiol, 24:*53-62.

Brown, IH (1959): Epilepsy in conjoined Siamese twins. *Electroenceph Clin Neurophysiol, 11:*565-570.

Brugge, JF (1965): An electroencephalographic study of the hippocampus and neocortex in unrestrained rats following septal lesions. *Electroenceph Clin Neurophysiol, 18:*36-44.

Bryson, D, and S Schacher (1969): Behavioral analysis of mammalian sleep and learning. *Perspect Biol Med, 12:*71-79.

Buendia, N, M Goode, G Sierra, and JP Segundo (1963): Responsiveness and discrimination during sleep. *Experientia, 19:*208-209.

Bulow, K, and DH Ingvar (1963): Respiration and electroencephalography in narcolepsy, *Neurol, 13:*321-326.

Caldwell, DF (1969): Differential levels of stage IV sleep in a group of clinically similar chronic schizophrenic patients. *Biol Psychiat, 1:*131-141.

Caldwell, DF, AJ Brane, and PGS Beckett (1970): Sleep patterns in normal and psychotic children. *Arch Gen Psychiat, 22:*500-503.

Caldwell, DF, and EF Domino (1967): Electroencephalographic and eye movement patterns during sleep in chronic schizophrenic patients. *Electroenceph Clin Neurophysiol, 22:*414-420.

Calvet, J, MC Calvet, and JM Langlois (1965): Diffuse cortical activation waves during so-called desynchronized EEG patterns. *J Neurophysiol, 28:* 893-907.

Carli, G, K Diete-Spiff, and O Pompeiano (1966): Presynaptic and postsynaptic inhibition of transmission and cutaneous afferent volleys through the cuneate nucleus during sleep. *Experientia, 22:*239-240.

Carli, G, K Diete-Spiff, and O Pompeiano (1967): Transmission of sensory information through the lemniscal pathway during sleep. *Arch Ital Biol, 105:* 31-51.

Carli, G and A Zanchetti (1965): A study of pontine lesions suppressing deep sleep in the cat. *Arch Ital Biol, 103:*751-787.

Carroll, D, SA Lewis, and I Oswald (1969): Effect of barbiturates on dreams content. *Nature, 223:*865-866.

Cartwright, RD, N Bernick, G Borowitz, and A Kling (1969): Effect of an erotic movie on sleep and dreams on young men. *Arch Gen Psychiat, 20:* 262-271.

Casati, C, N Dagnino, E Favale, M Manfredi, A Seitun, and A Targlione (1969): Functional changes of somatosensory system during deep sleep. *Electroenceph Clin Neurophysiol, 27:*289-295.

Castaldo, V (1968): Electroencephalographic study of sleep patterns of mongoloids as related to degree of mental retardation (abstract), *Psychophysiol, 5:* 213.

Castaldo, V, and PS Holzman (1967): The effect of hearing one's own voice on sleep mentation. *J Nerv Ment Dis, 144:*2-13.

Castaldo, V, and PS Holzman (1969): The effect of hearing one's own voice on dream content: a replication. *J Nerv Ment Dis, 148:*74-82.

Castaldo, V, and H Shevrin (1970): Different effect of an auditory stimulus as a function of rapid eye movement and non-rapid eye movement sleep. *J Nerv Ment Dis, 150:*195-200.

Catt, KJ (1970): Growth hormone. *Lancet, 1:*933-939.

Catton, B (1957): *A Stillness at Appomattox.* New York, Doubleday, p. 139.

Cayler, GG, J Mays, and HD Riley, Jr (1961): Cardiorespiratory syndrome of obesity (Pickwickian syndrome) in children. *Pediatrics, 27:237-245.*

Chin, JH, EK Killam, and KF Killam (1965): Factors affecting sensory input in the cat: Modification of evoked auditory potentials by reticular formation. *Electroenceph Clin Neurophysiol, 18:567-574.*

Clemente, CD, editor (1967): *Physiological Correlates of Dreaming.* New York, Academic Press. Reprinted as *Exp Neurol, Suppl 4,* 1967.

Clemes, SR, and WC Dement (1967): Effect of REM sleep deprivation on psychological functioning. *J Nerv Ment Dis, 144:485-491.*

Coccagna, G, M Mantovani, F Brignani, A Manzini, and E Lugaresi (1971): Arterial pressure changes during spontaneous sleep in man. *Electroenceph Clin Neurophysiol, 31:277-281.*

Cocks, JA (1967): Change in the concentration of lactic acid in the rat and hamster brain during natural sleep. *Nature, 215:1399-1400.*

Cohen, B, and M Feldman (1968): Relationship of electrical activity in pontine reticular formation and lateral geniculate body to rapid eye movements. *J Neurophysiol, 31:806-817.*

Cohen, HB, and WC Dement (1970): Prolonged tonic convulsions in REM deprived mice. *Brain Res, 22:421-422.*

Cohen, HB, RF Duncan, and WC Dement (1967): Sleep: The effect of electroconvulsive shock in cats deprived of REM sleep. *Science, 156:1646-1648.*

Cohen, HB, J Thomas, and WC Dement (1970): Sleep stages, REM deprivation and electroconvulsive threshold in the cat. *Brain Res, 19:317-321.*

Cooper, R, and A Hulme (1969): Changes of the EEG, intracranial pressure and other variables during sleep in patients with intracranial lesions. *Electroenceph Clin Neurophysiol, 27:12-22.*

Cordeau, JP, A Moreau, A Beaulnes, and C Lawrin (1963): EEG and behavioral changes following microinjections of acetylcholine and adrenaline in the brain stem of cats. *Arch Ital Biol, 101:30-47.*

Corletto, F, A Gentilomo, A Rosadini, GF Rossi, and J Zattoni (1967): Visual evoked responses during sleep in man. *Electroenceph Clin Neurophysiol, Suppl 26:61-69.*

Corvalan, JC (1969): Correlation of electroencephalographic, reaction time, and auditory thresholds on 24-hour recording (abstract). *Electroenceph Clin Neurophysiol, 27:696.*

Costin, A, and DR Hafemann (1970): Relationship between oculomotor nucleus and lateral geniculate body monophasic waves. *Experientia, 26:972.*

Coulter, JD, BK Lester, and HL Williams (1971): Reserpine and sleep. *Psychopharmacol, 19:134-147.*

Creutzfeld, O, and R Jung (1960): Neuronal discharge in the cats motor cortex during sleep and arousal. In Ciba Symposium, *The Nature of Sleep.* Boston, Little, Brown, pp. 131-170.

Dagnino, N, E Favale, C Loeb, M Manfredi, and A Seitun (1967): Nervous mechanisms underlying phasic changes in thalamic transmission during deep sleep. *Electroenceph Clin Neurophysiol, Suppl 26:*156-163.

Dagnino, N, E Favale, C Loeb, M Manfredi, and A Seitun (1969): Presynaptic and postsynaptic changes in specific thalamic nuclei during deep sleep. *Arch Ital Biol, 107:*668-684.

Dalton, A, and AH Black (1968): Hippocampal electrical activity during the operant conditioning of movement and refraining from movement. *Commun Behav Biol, 2:*267-273.

Daly, DD (1968): The effect of sleep upon the electroencephalogram in patients with brain tumors. *Electroenceph Clin Neurophysiol, 25:*521-529.

Daly, DD, and RE Yoss (1957): Electroencephalogram in narcolepsy. *Electroenceph Clin Neurophysiol, 9:*109-120.

Daly, RJ, and C Hassall (1970): Reported sleep on maintenance hemodialysis. *Brit Med J, 2:*508-509.

Davis, JM, WA Himwich, and M Stout (1969): Cerebral amino acids during deprivation of paradoxical sleep. *Biol Psychiat, 1:*387-390.

Davison, K, JP Duffy, and JW Osselton (1970): A comparison of sleep patterns in natural and mandrax- and tuinal-induced sleep. *Canad Med Assoc J, 102:* 506-508.

deJesus, PV Jr, and WS Masland (1970): The role of nasopharyngeal electrodes in clinical electroencephalography. *Neurol, 20:*869-878.

Dement, WC (1955): Dream recall and eye movement during sleep in schizophrenics and normals. *J Nerv Ment Dis, 122:*263-269.

Dement, WC (1964): Eye movements during sleep. In Bender, MB (editor): *The Oculomotor System.* New York, Harper and Row, pp. 366-416.

Dements, WC (1966): Discussion. *Amer J Psychiat, 123:*136-142.

Dement, WC (1967): Possible physiological determinants of a possible dream-intensity cycle. *Exp Neurol Suppl, 4:*38-56.

Dement, WC (1969): The biological role of REM sleep (circa 1968). In Kales, A (editor): *Sleep: Physiology and Pathology.* Philadelphia, Lippincott, pp. 245-265.

Dement, WC, and C Fisher (1963): Experimental interference with the sleep cycle. *Canad Psychiat Assoc J, 8:*400-405.

Dement, WC, S Greenberg, and R Klein (1966): The effect of partial REM sleep deprivation and delayed recovery. *J Psychiat Res, 4:*141-152.

Dement, WC, E Kahn, and HP Roffwarg (1965): The influence of the laboratory situation on the dreams of the experimental subject. *J Nerv Ment Dis, 140:*119-131.

Dement, WC, and N Kleitman (1957): Cyclic variations in EEG during sleep and their relation to eye movements, body mobility, and dreaming. *Electroenceph Clin Neurophysiol, 9:*673-690.

Dement, WC, and N Kleitman (1957): The relation of eye movements during sleep to dream activity: an objective method for the study of dreaming. *J Exp Psychol, 53:*339-346.

Dement, WC, A Rechtschaffen, and G Gulevich (1966): The nature of the narcoleptic sleep attack. *Neurol, 16*:18-33.

Dement, WC, and EA Wolpert (1958): The relation of eye movements, body motility, and external stimuli to dream content. *J Exp Psychol, 55*:543-553.

Desiraju, T, BK Anand, and B Singh (1966): Electrographic studies on the nature of sleep and wakefulness. *Physiol Behav, 1*:285-291.

Desmedt, JE, and J Manil (1970): Somatosensory evoked potentials of the normal human neonate in REM sleep, in slow wave sleep and in waking. *Electroenceph Clin Neurophysiol, 29*:113-518.

Dexter, JD, and ED Weitzman (1970): The relationship of nocturnal headaches to sleep stage patterns. *Neurol, 20*:513-518.

Dewan, EM (1969): The programming (P) hypothesis for REMS. *US Air Force Technical Report* AFCRL-69-0298, Hanscom Field, Massachusetts.

Dewan, EM (1970): The programming (P) hypothesis for REM sleep. *Int Psychiat Clinics, 7*:295-307.

Diaz-Guerrero, R, JS Gottlieb, and JR Knott, (1946): The sleep of patients with manic-depressive psychosis, depressive type. *Psychosomatic Med, 8:* 399-404.

Domhoff, B, and J Kamiya (1964a): Problems in dream content study with objective indicators. I. A comparison of home and laboratory dream reports. *Arch Gen Psychiat, 11*:519-524.

Domhoff, B, and J Kamiya (1964b): Problems in dream content study with objective indicators: II Appearance of experimental situation in laboratory dream narratives. *Arch Gen Psychiat, 11*:525-528.

Domhoff, B, and J Kamiya (1964c): Problems in dream content study with objective indicators: III. Changes in dream content throughout the night. *Arch Gen Psychiat, 11*:529-532.

Domino, EF, and M Stawiski (1971): Modification of the cat sleep cycle by hemicholinium-3, a cholinergic antisynthesis agent. *Res Commun Chem Pathol Physiol, 2*:461-467.

Drachman, DB, and RJ Gumnit (1962): Periodic alteration of consciousness in the "Pickwickian" syndrome. *Arch Neurol, 6*:471-477.

Dreyfus-Brisac, C (1970): Ontogenesis of sleep in human prematures after 32 weeks of conceptual age. *Develop Psychobiol, 3*:91-121.

Dreyfus-Brisac, C and N Monod (1970): Sleeping behaviour in abnormal newborn infants. *Neuropadiatrie, 3*:354-366.

Drucker-Colin, RR, JA Rojas-Ramirez, J Vera-Trueba, G Monroy-Avala, and R Hernandez-Peon (1970): Effect of crossed-perfusion of the midbrain reticular formation upon sleep. *Brain Res, 23*:269-273.

Duffy, JP and K Davison (1968): A female case of the Kleine-Levin syndrome. *Brit J Psychiat, 114*:77-84.

Dunleavy, DLF, AW MacLean, and I Oswald (1971): Debrisoquine, guanethidine, propanolol and human sleep. *Psychopharmacol, 21*:101-110.

Dunlop, CW, and MD Waks (1968): Effects of arousal state on click responses in the cat cochlear nucleus. *J Audit Res, 8*:97-110.

Eason, RG, P Groves, CT White, and D Oden (1967): Evoked cortical potentials: relation to visual field and handedness. *Science, 156:*1643-1646.

Eccles, JC (1961): Discussion. In Ciba Symposium, *The Nature of Sleep.* Boston, Little, Brown, p. 384.

Editorial (1965): Norbert Weiner, 1894-1964. *J Nerv Ment Dis, 140:*3.

Ekbom, K (1966): Familial multiple schlerosis associated with narcolepsy. *Arch Neurol, 15:*337-344.

Elian, M, and B Bornstein (1969): The Kleine-Levin syndrome with intermittent abnormality in the EEG. *Electroenceph Clin Neurophysiol, 27:*601-604.

Elliott, FA (1971): *Clinical Neurology,* 2nd ed. Philadelphia, Saunders.

Empson, JAC, and PRF Clarke (1970): Rapid eye movements and remembering. *Nature, 227:*287-288.

Ephron, HS, and P Carrington (1966): Rapid eye movement sleep and cortical homeostasis. *Psychol Rev, 73:*500-526.

Epstein, AW, (1967): Body image alterations during seizures and dreams of epileptics. *Arch Neurol, 16:*613-619.

Epstein, AW, and W Hill (1966): Ictal phenomena during REM sleep of a temporal lobe epileptic. *Arch Neurol, 15:*367-375.

Evans, FJ, LA Gustafson, DN O'Connell, MT Orne, and RE Shor (1966): Response during sleep with intervening waking amnesia. *Science, 152:*666-667.

Evans, FJ, LA Gustafson, DN O'Connell, MT Orne, and RE Shor (1969): Sleep-induced behavioral response: Relationship to susceptibility to hypnosis and laboratory sleep patterns. *J Nerv Ment Dis, 148:*467-476.

Evans, FJ, LA Gustafson, DN O'Connell, MT Orne, and RE Shor (1970): Verbally induced behavioral responses during sleep. *J Nerv Ment Dis, 150:* 171-187.

Evans, JI, and SA Lewis (1968): Drug withdrawl state: an EEG sleep study. *Arch Gen Psychiat, 19:*631-634.

Evans, JI, AW MacLean, AAA Ismail, and D Love (1971): Concentrations of plasma testosterone in normal men during sleep. *Nature, 229:*261-262.

Evans, JI, and O Ogunremi (1970): Sleep and hypnotics: further experiments. *Brit Med J, 3:*310-313.

Evans, JI, and I Oswald (1966): Some experiments in the chemistry of narcoleptic sleep. *Brit J Psychiat, 112:*401-404.

Evarts, EV (1960): Effects of sleep and waking on activity of single units in the unrestrained cat. In Ciba Symposium, *The Nature of Sleep,* Boston, Little, Brown, pp. 171-187.

Evarts, EV (1962): Activity of neurons in visual cortex of the cat during sleep with low voltage fast activity. *J Neurophysiol, 25:*812-816.

Evarts, EV (1964): Temporal patterns of discharge of pyramidal tract neurons during sleep and waking in the monkey. *J Neurophysiol, 27:*152-171.

Evarts, EV (1965): Relation of cell size to effects of sleep in pyramidal tract neurons, *Prog Brain Res, 18:*81-91.

Evarts, EV (1969): Neuronal activity during wakefulness and sleep: Some comments. *Biol Psychiat, 1:*143-145.

Favale, E, C Loeb, M Manfredi, and G Sacco (1965): Somatic afferent transmission and cortical responsiveness during natural sleep and arousal in the cat. *Electroenceph Clin Neurophysiol, 18:*354-368.

Feinberg, I, M Braun, RL Koresko, and F Gottlieb (1969a): Stage 4 sleep in schizophrenia. *Arch Gen Psychiat, 21:*262-266.

Feinberg, I, M Braun, and E Shulman (1969b): EEG sleep patterns in mental retardation. *Electroenceph Clin Neurophysiol, 27:*128-141.

Feinberg, I and EV Evarts (1969): Some implications of sleep research for psychiatry. In J Zubin and C Shagass (editors): *Neurobiological Aspects of Psychopathology.* New York, Grune and Stratton, pp. 334-393.

Feinberg, I, RL Koresko, N Heller, and HR Steinberg (1965a): Unusually high dream time in a hallucinating patient. *Amer J Psychiat, 121:*1018-1020.

Feinberg, I, RL Koresko, and IR Schaffner (1965b): Sleep electroencephalographic and eye movement patterns in patients with chronic brain syndrome. *J Psychiat Res, 3:*11-26.

Feinberg, I, PH Wender, RL Koresko, F Gottlieb, and JA Piehuta (1969a): Differential effects of chlorpromazine and phenobarbital on EEG sleep patterns. *J Psychiat Res, 7:*101-109.

Feldman, MH (1971): Physiological observations in a chronic case of "locked-in" syndrome. *Neurol, 21:*459-478.

Findlay, ALR, and JN Hayward (1969): Spontaneous activity of single neurones in the hypothalamus of rabbits during sleep and waking. *J Physiol (London), 201:*237-258.

Finley, WW (1971): An EEG study of the sleep of enuretics at three age levels. *Clin Electroenceph, 2:*35-39.

Firth, H, SA Lewis, OO Ogunremi, and I Oswald (1970): The effect of acute administration of (meta trifluoromethylphenyl)-1-(benzoyl oxy) ethyl amino-2-propane (780 SE) and fenfluramine on human sheep. *Brit J Pharmacol, 39:*462-463.

Fishbein, W (1970): Interference with conversion of memory from short-term to long-term storage by partial sleep deprivation. *Comm Behav Biol, 5:* 171-175.

Fishbein, W (1971): Disruptive effects of rapid eye movement sleep deprivation on long-term storage. *Physiol Behav, 6:*279-282.

Fisher, C, J Byrne, A Edwards, and E Kahn (1970): A psychophysiological study of nightmares. *J Amer Psychoanalyt Assoc, 18:*747-782.

Fisher, C, J Gross, and J Zulch (1965): Cycle of penile erections synchronous with dreaming (REM) sleep: preliminary report. *Arch Gen Psychiat, 12:* 29-45.

Florio, W, A Scotti de Carolis, and VG Longo (1968): Observations on the effect of DL-parachlorophenylalanine on the electroencephalogram. *Physiol Behav, 3:*861-863.

Foulkes, D (1962): Dream reports from different stages of sleep. *J Abn Soc Psychol, 65:*14-25.

Foulkes, D (1966): *The Psychology of Sleep.* New York, Scribner.

Foulkes, D, JD Larson, EM Swanson, and M Rardin (1969): Two studies of childhood dreaming. *Amer J Orthopsychiat, 39:*627-643.

Foulkes, D, RT Pivik, JB Aherns, and EM Swanson (1968): Effects of "dream deprivation" on dream content: An attempted cross night replication. *J Abn Psychol, 73:*403-415.

Foulkes, D, and G Vogel (1965): Mental activity at sleep onset. *J Abn Psychol, 70:*231-243.

Frank, GS, and GV Pegram (1970): Interrelations of sleep and focal epileptiform discharge in monkeys with alumina creme lesions. *US Air Force Technical Report ARL-TR-70-12.*

Franklin, LM (1969): Sleep and hypnotics in a psychiatric admission ward. *New Zealand Med J, 69:*353-355.

Fredrickson, CJ, and JA Hobson (1970): Electrical stimulation of the brain stem and subsequent sleep. *Arch Ital Biol, 108:*564-576.

Freedman, A, L Luborsky, and RB Harvey (1970): Dream time (REM) and psychotherapy. *Arch Gen Psychiat, 22:*33-39.

Freemon, FR (1970): Reciprocal environmental surveillance model of sleep. *J Theor Biol, 27:*339-340.

Freemon, FR, HW Agnew, Jr, and BJ Wilder (1970): Electrical activity of human midbrain and hypothalamus during sleep. *Comprehen Psychiat, 11:* 356-360.

Freemon, FR, HW Agnew, Jr, and RL Williams (1965): An electroencephalographic study of the effects of meprobamate on human sleep. *Clin Pharmacol Therapy, 6:*172-176.

Freemon, FR, and FT Drake (1967): Abnormal emotional reactions to hospitalization jeopardizing medical treatment. *Psychosomatics, 8:*150-155.

Freemon, FR, DW Goodwin, JA Halikas, and E Othmer (1971): An electroencephalographic study of memory loss during alcoholic intoxication. *Dis Nerv Syst, 32:*848-852.

Freemon, FR, JJ McNew, and WR Adey (1969): Sleep of unrestrained chimpanzee: cortical and subcortical recordings. *Exp Neurol, 25:*129-137.

Freemon, FR, JJ McNew, and WR Adey (1970): Sleep of unrestrained chimpanzee: differences between first and last rapid eye movement periods. *Folia Primatol, 13:*144-149.

Freemon, FR, JJ McNew, and WR Adey (1971): Chimpanzee sleep stages. *Electroenceph Clin Neurophysiol, 31:*485-489.

Freemon, FR, and RD Walter (1970): Electrical activity of human limbic system during sleep. *Comprehen Psychiat, 11:*544-551.

French, JD (1952): Brain lesions associated with prolonged unconsciousness. *Arch Neurol Psychiat, 68:*727-740.

French, JD, and HW Magoun (1952): Effects of chronic lesions in central cephalic brain stem of monkeys. *Arch Neurol Psychiat, 68:*591-604.

Freud, S (1900): *The Interpretation of Dreams.*

Friedlander, WJ (1952): Alterations of basal ganglion tremor during sleep. *Neurol, 2:*222-225.

Friedman, RC, JT Bigger, and DS Kornfeld (1971): The intern and sleep loss. *New Engl J Med, 285*:201-203.

Friend, DG (1969): Generic terminology and the cost of drugs. *J Amer Med Assoc, 209*:80-84.

Fromm, E (1951): *The Forgotten Language.* New York, Rinehart.

Frommer, G, and R Galambos (1964): Arousal effects of specific thalamocortical evoked responses (abstract). *Fed Proceed, 23*:209.

Gaarder, K (1966): A conceptual model of sleep. *Arch Gen Psychiat, 14*: 253-260.

Gambi, D, FM Ferro, and S Mazza (1970): Analysis of sleep in progressive myoclonus epilepsy. *Europ Neurol, 3*:347-364.

Ganado, W (1958): The narcolepsy syndrome. *Neurol, 8*:487-496.

Gardner, R, and ED Weitzman (1967): Examination for optokinetic nystagmus in sleep and waking. *Arch Neurol, 16*:415-420.

Garland, H, D Sumner, and P Fourman (1965): The Kleine-Levin syndrome: some further observations. *Neurol, 15*:1161-1167.

Gassel, MM, PL Marchiafava, and O Pompeiano (1965): Activity of the red nucleus during desynchronized sleep in unrestrained cats. *Arch Ital Biol, 103*:369-396.

Gastaut, H, E Lugaresi, G Berti Ceroni, and G Coccagna (1968) editors, *The Abnormalities of Sleep in Man.* Bologna, Aulo Gaggi.

Geller, MR, N Gourdji, N Christoff, and E Fox (1969): The effects of sleep deprivation on the EEGs of epileptic children. *Develop Med Child Neurol, 11*:771-776.

Giannazzo, E, T Manzoni, R Raffaele, S Sapienza, and A Urbano (1968): Changes in the sleep-wakefulness cycle induced by chronic fastigial lesions in the cat. *Brain Res, 11*:281-284.

Gibbs, EL, and FA Gibbs (1947): Sleep records in epilepsy. *Res Publ Assoc Res Nerv Ment Dis, 26*:366-372.

Glick, BS, D Schulman, and S Turecki (1971): Diazepam (Valium) treatment in childhood sleep disorders. *Dis Nerv Syst, 32*:565-566.

Globus, GG (1966): Rapid eye movement cycle in real time. *Arch Gen Psychiat, 15*:654-659.

Globus, GG (1969): A syndrome associated with sleeping late. *Psychosom Med, 6*:528-535.

Goff, WR, T Allison, and BS Rosner (1966): Cerebral somatosensory responses evoked during sleep in man. *Electroenceph Clin Neurophysiol, 21*:1-9.

Goldie, L, JAH Curtis, U Svendsen, and NRC Robertson (1968): Abnormal sleep rhythms in mongol babies. *Lancet, 1*:229-230.

Goldie, L, and C Van Velzer (1965): Innate sleep rhythms. *Brain, 88*:1043-1056.

Goldring, S, E Aras, and PC Weber (1970): Comparative study of sensory input to motor cortex in animals and man. *Electroenceph Clin Neurophysiol, 29*:537-550.

Goodall, J (1962): Nest building behavior in the free ranging chimpanzee. *Ann NY Acad Sci, 102*:445-467.

Goodall, J (1963): My life among wild chimpanzees. *Nat Geogr, 124*:272-308.

Goodenough, DR, HB Lewis, A Shapiro, and I Slesler (1965): Some correlates of dream reporting following laboratory awakenings. *J Nerv Ment Dis, 140:* 365-373.

Goodenough, DR, A Shapiro, M Holden, and L Steinschriber (1959): A comparison of "dreamers" and "non dreamers": eye movements, electroencephalograms, and the recall of dreams. *J Abn Soc Psychol, 59*:295-302.

Goodwin, DW, FR Freemon, BM Ianzito, and E Othmer (1970): Alcohol and narcolepsy. *Brit J Psychiat, 117*:705-706.

Gowers, WR (1907): *The Border-Land of Epilepsy.*

Grastyan, E, G Karmos, L Vereczkey, and L Kellenyi (1966): The hippocampal electrical correlates of the homoeostatic regulation of motivation. *Electroenceph Clin Neurophysiol, 21*:34-53.

Grastyan, E, K Lissak, I Madarasz, and H Donhoffer (1959): Hippocampal electrical activity during the development of conditioned reflexes. *Electroenceph Clin Neurophysiol, 11*:409-430.

Gramsbergen, A, P Schwartze, and HFR Prechtl (1970): The postnatal development of sleep in the rat. *Develop Psychobiol, 3*:267-280.

Granit, R (1968): The development of retinal physiology. *Science, 160*:1192-1196.

Green, WJ (1965): The effect of LSD on the sleep-dream cycle. *J Nerv Ment Dis, 140*:417-426.

Green, WJ (1969): LSD and the sleep-dream cycle. *Exp Med Surg, 27*:138-144.

Greenberg, R (1970): Dreaming and memory. *Int Psychiat Clinics, 7*:258-267.

Greenberg, R, D Mahler, and C Pearlman (1969): Dreaming and nitrous oxide. *Arch Gen Psychiat, 21*:691-695.

Greenberg, R, and C Pearlman (1967): Delirium tremens and dreaming. *Amer J Psychiat, 124*:133-142.

Greenberg, R, and C Pearlman (1968): Sleep patterns in temporal lobe epilepsy. *Comprehen Psychiat, 9*:194-199.

Greenberg, R, C Pearlman, R Brooks, R Mayer, and E Hartmann (1968): Dreaming and Korsakov's psychosis. *Arch Gen Psychiat, 18*:203-209.

Greenberg, R, C Pearlman, R Fingar, J Kantrowitz, and S Kawlicke (1970): The effects of dream deprivation: Implications for a theory of the psychological function of dreaming. *Brit J Med Psychol, 43*:1-11.

Gresham, SC, HW Agnew Jr, and RL Williams (1965): The sleep of depressed patients. *Arch Gen Psychiat, 13*:503-507.

Gresham, SC, WB Webb, and RL Williams (1963): Alcohol and caffeine: effect on inferred visual dreaming. *Science, 140*:1226-1227.

Grinspoon, L (1971): Marihuana. *Int J Psychiat, 9*:488-512.

Gross, J, J Byrne, and C Fisher (1965): Eye movements during emergent stage 1 EEG in subjects with lifelong blindness. *J Nerv Ment Dis, 141*:365-370.

Gross, M, D Goodenough, M Tobin, E Halpert, D Leport, A Perlstein, M Serota, J Debeanco, R Fuller, and I Kishner (1966): Sleep disturbance and hallucinations in the acute alcoholic psychoses. *J Nerv Ment Dis, 142:*493-514.

Grosser, GS, and AW Siegal (1971): Emergence of a tonic-phasic model for sleep and dreaming: behavioral and physiological observations. *Psychol Bull, 75:*60-72.

Guerrero-Figueroa, R, and RG Health (1964): Evoked responses and changes during attentive factors in man. *Arch Neurol, 10:*74-78.

Gulevich, G, WC Dement, and L Johnson (1966): Psychiatric and EEG observations on a case of prolonged (264 hours) wakefulness. *Arch Gen Psychiat, 15:*29-35.

Gulevich, GD, WC Dement, and VP Zarcone (1967): All-night sleep recordings of chronic schizophrencis in remission. *Comprehen Psychiat, 8:*141-159.

Haider, I (1968): Patterns of insomnia in depressive illness: subjective evaluation. *Brit J Psychiat, 114:*1127-1132.

Haider, I (1969): Effects of a nonbarbiturate hypnotic (nitrazepam-Mogadon) on human sleep: an electroencephalographic study. *Pakistan Medical Forum, 4:*13-28.

Haider, I, and I Oswald (1971): Effects of amylobarbitone and nitrazepam on the electrodermogram and other features of sleep. *Brit J Psychiat, 118:*519-522.

Hall, CS (1953): *The Meaning of Dreams.* New York, Harper.

Hambert, O, and I Petersen (1970); Clinical, electroencephalographical and neuropharmacological studies in syndromes of progressive myoclonus epilepsy. *Acta Neurol Scandinav, 46:*149-186.

Hammond, WA (1883): *Sleep and Its Derangements.* Philadelphia, Lippincott.

Hartmann, E (1965): The D state: a review and discussion of studies on the physiologic state concomitant with dreaming. *New Eng J Med, 273:*30-35, 87-92.

Hartmann, E (1966): Reserpine: its effect on the sleep-dream cycle in man. *Psychopharmacol, 9:*242-247.

Hartmann, E (1967a): The effect of l-tryptophan on the sleep-dream cycle in man. *Psychon Sci, 8:*479-480.

Hartmann, E (1967b): *The Biology of Dreaming.* Springfield, Thomas.

Hartmann, E (1968a): The 90-minute sleep dream cycle. *Arch Gen Psychiat, 18:*280-286.

Hartmann, E (1968b): The effect of four drugs on sleep patterns in man. *Psychopharmacol, 12:*346-353.

Hartmann, E (1968c): Longitudinal studies of sleep and dream patterns in manic-depressive patients. *Arch Gen Psychiat, 19:*312-329

Hartmann, E (1970): The D-state and norepinephine-dependent systems. In E Hartmann (editor): *Sleep and Dreaming.* Boston, Little, Brown, pp. 308-328.

Hartmann, E., editor (1970): *Sleep and Dreaming.* Boston, Little, Brown.

Hartmann, E, F Baekeland, G Zwilling, and P Hoy (1971): Sleep need: How much sleep and what kind? *Amer J Psychiat, 127:*1001-1008.

Hartmann, E, R Chung, and C Chien (1971): L-tryptophane and sleep. *Psychopharmacol, 19*:114-127.

Hassin, GB (1951): Nocturnal dysesthesias: Schultze-Wartenberg syndrome. *J Neuropath Clin Neurol, 1*:320-324.

Haulica, I, L Abalei, C Teodorescu, V Rosca, A Haulica, M Moisiu, and C Haller (1970): The influence of deprivation of paradoxical sleep on cerebral ammonia metabolism. *J Neurochem, 17*:823-826.

Hauri, P (1970): Evening activity, sleep mentation, and subjective sleep quality. *J Abn Psychol, 76*:270-275.

Hawkins, DR, and J Mendels (1966): Sleep disturbance in depressive syndromes. *Amer J Psychiat, 123*:682-690.

Hayden, MP (1969): Sleep onset REM in normals (abstract). *Electroenceph Clin Neurophysiol, 27*:685.

Hays, HR (1963): *In the Beginnings: Early Man and His Gods.* New York, Putnam.

Hazra, J (1970): Effects of hemicholinium-3 on slow wave and paradoxical sleep of cat. *Europ J Pharmacol, 11*:395-397.

Hellman, L, F Nakada, J Curti, ED Weitzman, J Kream, H Roffwarg, S Ellman, DK Fukushima, and TF Gallagher (1970): Cortisol is secreted episodically by normal man. *J Clin Endocrinol Metab, 30*:411-422.

Heninger, GR, RK McDonald, WR Goff, and A Sollberger (1969): Diurnal variations in the cerebral evoked response and EEG: relations to 17-hydroxycorticosteroid levels. *Arch Neurol, 21*:330-337.

Hernandez-Peon, R (1965): A neurophysiologic model of dreams and hallucinations. *J Nerv Ment Dis, 141*:623-650.

Hernandez-Peon, R, G Chavez-Ibarra, PJ Morgane, and C Timo-Iara (1963): Limbic cholinergic pathways involved in sleep and emotional behavior. *Exp Neurol, 8*:93-111.

Hernandez-Peon, R, JJ O'Flaherty, and AL Mazzuchelli-O'Flaherty (1965): Modifications of tactile evoked potentials at the spinal trigeminal sensory nucleus during wakefulness and sleep. *Exp Neurol, 13*:40-57.

Hernandez-Peon, R, JJ O'Flaherty, and AL Mazzuchelli-O'Flaherty (1967): Sleep and other behavioral effects induced by acetylcholinic stimulation of basal temporal cortex and stirate structures. *Brain Res, 4*:243-267.

Hery, F, JF Pujol, M Lopez, J Macon, and J Glowinski (1970): Increased synthesis and utilization of serotonin in the central nervous system of the rat during paradoxical sleep deprivation. *Brain Res, 21*:391-403.

Hess, WR (1954): The diencephalic sleep centre. In J.F. Delafresnaye (editor): *Brain Mechanisms and Consciousness.* Springfield, Thomas, pp. 117-125.

Hess, WR (1956): *Hypothalamus and Thalamus.* Stuttgart, Verlag, p. 22.

Hishikawa, Y, and Z Kaneko (1965): Electroencephalographic study of narcolepsy. *Electroenceph Clin Neurophysiol, 18*:249-259.

Hishikawa, Y, H Nan'no, M Tachibana, E Furuya, H Koida, and Z Kaneko (1968): The nature of sleep attack and other symptoms of narcolepsy. *Electroenceph Clin Neurophysiol, 24*:1-10.

Hishikawa, Y, N Sumitsuji, K Matsumoto, and Z Kaneko (1965): H-reflex and EMG of the mental and hyoid muscles during sleep, with special reference to narcolepsy. *Electroenceph Clin Neurophysiol, 18:*487-492.

Hobson, JA (1969): Sleep: biochemical aspects. *New Engl J Med, 281:*1468-1470.

Hobson, JA (1970): Brainstem signs, sleep attacks, and REM sleep enhancement (abstract). *Psychophysiol, 7:*310.

Hobson, JA, J Alexander, and CJ Frederickson (1969): The effect of lateral geniculate lesions on phasic electrical activity of the cortex during desynchronized sleep in the cat. *Brain Res, 14:*607-621.

Hobson, JA, F Goldfrank, and F Snyder (1965): Respiration and mental activity in sleep. *J Psychiat Res, 3:*79-90.

Hobson, JA, and RW McCarley (1970): Spontaneous unit activity of cat cerebellar Purkinje cells in sleep and waking (abstract). *Psychophysiol, 7:*311.

Hobson, JA, and RW McCarley (1971a): Cortical unit activity in sleep and waking. *Electroencephal Clin Neurophysiol, 30:*97-112.

Hobson, JA, and RW McCarley (1971b): *Neuronal Activity in Sleep: An Annotated Bibliography.* Los Angeles, UCLA Brain Information Service Publications.

Hodes, R, and WC Dement (1964): Depression of electrically induced reflexes ("H-reflexes") in man during low voltage EEG "sleep." *Electroenceph Clin Neurophysiol, 17:*617-629.

Hodes, R, and JI Suzuki (1965): Comparative thresholds of cortex, vestibular system and reticular formation in wakefulness, sleep and rapid eye movement periods. *Electroenceph Clin Neurophysiol, 18:*239-248.

Hoffman, JS, and EF Domino (1969): Comparative effects of reserpine on the sleep cycle of man and cat. *J Pharmacol Exp Therap, 170:*190-198.

Hunter, R, W Blackwood, and J Bull (1968): Three cases of frontal meningiomas presenting psychiatrically. *Brit Med J, 3:*9-16.

Hurwitz, LJ, SN Groch, IS Wright, and FH McDowell (1959): Carotid artery occlusive syndrome. *Arch Neurol, 1:*491-501.

Huttenlocher, PR (1960): Effects of state of arousal on click responses in the mesencephalic reticular formation. *Electroenceph Clin Neurophysiol, 12:*819-827.

Huttenlocher, PR (1961): Evoked and spontaneous activity in single units of medial brain stem during natural sleep and waking. *J Neurophysiol, 24:*451-468.

Irvine, DRF, WR Webster, and KH Sack (1970): Effects of repetitive stimulation and state of arousal on cochlear potentials. *Exp Neurol, 29:*16-30.

Iskander, TN, and R Kaebling (1970): Catecholamines, a dream sleep model, and depression. *Amer J Psychiat, 127:*43-50.

Itil, TM (1969): Digital computer "sleep prints" and psychopharmacology. *Biol Psychiat, 1:*91-95.

Itil, TM (1970): Digital computer analysis of the electroencephalogram during rapid eye movement sleep state in man. *J Nerv Ment Dis, 150:*201-208.

Iwama, K, T Kawamoto, H Sakakura, and T Kasamatsu (1966): Responsiveness of cat lateral geniculate at pre- and postsynaptic levels during natural sleep. *Physiol Behav, 1:*43-53.

Iwamura, Y, Y Uchino, and S Ozawa (1967): Parasympathetic activity during para-sleep. *Proc Jap Acad Sci, 43:*352-354.

Jacobs, BL, and DJ McGinty (1971): Amygdala unit activity during sleep and waking. *Exp Neurol, 33:*1-15.

Jacobs, L, M Feldman, and MB Bender (1971a): Eye movements during sleep: I. The pattern in the normal human. *Arch Neurol, 25:*151-159.

Jacobs, L, M Feldman, and MB Bender (1971b): Eye movements during sleep: II. The pattern with upward gaze paralysis. *Arch Neurol, 25:*212-217.

Jacobson, A, A Kales, D Lehmann, and FS Hoedemaker (1964): Muscle tonus in human subjects during sleep and waking. *Exp Neurol, 10:*418-424.

Jacobson, A, A Kales, D Lehmann, and JR Zweizig (1965): Somnambulism: all-night electroencephalographic studies. *Science, 148:*975-977.

Jasper, HH, and J Tessier (1971): Acetylcholine liberation from cerebral cortex during paradoxical (REM) sleep. *Science, 172:*601-602.

Jeannerod, M, and K Sakai (1970): Occipital and geniculate potentials related to eye movements in the unanesthetized cat. *Brain Res, 19:*361-377.

Johns, MW (1971): Methods for assessing human sleep. *Arch Intern Med, 127:*484-492.

Johns, MW, P Egan, TJA Gay, and JP Masterton (1970): Sleep habits and symptoms in male medical and surgical patients. *Brit Med J, 2:*509-512.

Johnson, J, and AD Clift (1968): Dependence on hypnotic drugs in general practice. *Brit Med J, 2:*613-617.

Johnson, LC, JA Burdick, and J Smith (1970): Sleep during alcohol intake and withdrawal in the chronic alcoholic. *Arch Gen Psychiat, 22:*406-418.

Johnson, LC, and W Karpan (1968): Autonomic correlates of the spontaneous K-complex. *Psychophysiol, 4:*444-452.

Jones, HS, and I Oswald (1968): Two cases of healthy insomnia. *Electroenceph Clin Neurophysiol, 24:*378-380.

Jones, RM (1970): *The New Psychology of Dreaming.* New York, Grune Stratton.

Jouvet, M (1961): Telencephalic and rhombencephalic sleep in the cat. In Ciba Symposium: *The Nature of Sleep.* London, Churchill, pp. 188-206.

Jouvet, M (1962): Recherches sur les structures nerveuses et les mecanismes responsables des differentes phases du sommeil physiologique. *Arch Ital Biol, 100:*125-206.

Jouvet, M, editor, (1965): *Aspects Anatomo-Fonctionnels de la Physiologie du Sommeil.* Lyon, CNRS.

Jouvet, M (1967): Neurophysiology of the states of sleep. *Physiol Rev, 47:* 117-177.

Jouvet, M (1968): Insomnia and decrease of cerebral 5-hydroxytryptamine after destruction of the raphe system in the cat. *Adv Pharmacol, 6:*265-279.

Jouvet, M (1969): Biogenic amines and the states of sleep. *Science, 163*:32-41.

Jouvet, M (1972): Neurohumoral mechanisms regulating the sleep-waking cycle. In Olga Petre-Quadens (editor): *Basic Sleep Mechanisms,* in press.

Jouvet, M, P Bobillier, JF Pujol, and J Renault (1966): Effets des lesions du systeme du raphe sur le sommeil et la serotonine cerebrale. *Compt Rend Soc Biol, 160*:2343-2346.

Jouvet, M, F Michel, and D Mounier (1960): Analyse electroencephalographique chez le chat et chez l'homme. *Rev Neurol, 103*:189-205.

Jouvet, M, F Michel, and D Mounier (1960): Comparative study of the "paradoxical phase" of sleep in cat and man (abstract). *Electroenceph Clin Neurophysiol, 12*:937.

Jouvet-Mounier, D, L Astic, and D Lacote (1970): Ontogenesis of the states of sleep in rat, cat, and guinea pig during the first postnatal month. *Develop Psychobiol, 2*:216-239.

Jung, R and W Kuhlo (1965): Neurophysiological studies of abnormal night sleep and the Pickwickian syndrome. *Prog Brain Res, 18*:140-159.

Jurko, MF, and OJ Andy (1965): Serial EEG study following thalamotomy. *Electroenceph Clin Neurophysiol, 18*:500-503.

Kahn, M, BL Baker, and JM Weiss (1968): Treatment of insomnia by relaxation training. *J Abn Psychol, 6*:556-558.

Kahn, E, WC Dement, C Fisher, and JE Barmack (1962): Incidence of color in immediately recalled dreams. *Science, 137*:1054-1055.

Kahn, E, and C Fisher (1969): The sleep characteristics of the normal aged male. *J Nerv Ment Dis, 148*:477-494.

Kahn, E, C Fisher, J Byrne, A Edwards, D Davis, and A Frosch (1970): The influence of Valium, Thorazine, and Dilantin on stage 4 nightmares (abstract). *Psychophysiol, 7*:350.

Kahn, E, C Fisher, and L Lieberman (1970): Sleep characteristics of the human aged female. *Comprehen Psychiat, 11*:274-278.

Kajtor, F, J Hullay, L Farago, and K Haberland (1957): Effect of barbiturate sleep on the electrical activity of the hippocampus of patients with temporal lobe epilepsy. *Electroenceph Clin Neurophysiol, 9*:441-451.

Kales, A, editor (1969): *Sleep: Physiology and Pathology.* Philadelphia, Lippincott.

Kales, A, GL Adams, and JT Pearlman (1970a): Rapid eye movement (REM) sleep in ophthalmic patients. *Amer J Ophthalmol, 69*:615-622.

Kales, A, C Allen, MB Scharf, and JD Kales (1970b): Hynotic drugs and their effectiveness. *Arch Gen Psychiat, 23*:226-232.

Kales, A, C Allen, M Scharf, and TA Preston (1970c): Methodologic considerations and recommendations for sleep laboratory drug evaluation studies (abstract). *Psychopharmacol, 7*:344.

Kales, A, RD Ansel, CH Markham, MB Scharf, and TL Tan (1971): Sleep in patients with Parkinson's disease and normal subjects prior to and following levodopa administration. *Clin Pharmacol Therap, 12*:397-406.

Kales, A, GN Beall, RJ Berger, G Heuser, A Jacobson, JD Kales, AH Parmalee Jr, and RD Walter (1968): Sleep and dreams: recent research on clinical aspects. *Ann Int Med, 68*:1078-1104.

Kales, A, G Heuser, A Jacobson, JD Kales, J Hanley, JR Zweizig, and MJ Paulson (1967): All-night sleep studies in hypothyroid patients, before and after treatment. *J Clin Endocrinol, 27*:1593-1599.

Kales, A, FS Hoedemaker, A Jacobson, JD Kales, MJ Paulson, and TE Wilson (1967): Mentation during sleep: REM and NREM recall reports. *Percept Motor Skills, 24*:555-560.

Kales, A, A Jacobson, MJ Paulson, JD Kales, and RD Walter (1966): Somnambulism: psychophysiological correlates: I. All-night EEG studies. *Arch Gen Psychiat, 14*:586-594.

Kales, A and JD Kales (1970): Evaluation, diagnosis, and treatment of clinical conditions related to sleep. *J Amer Med Assoc, 213*:2229-2235.

Kales, A, JD Kales, MB Scharf and TL Tan (1970d) Hypnotics and altered sleep-dream patterns II: all-night EEG studies of chloral hydrate, flurazepam, and methaqualone. *Arch Gen Psychiat, 23*:219-225.

Kales, A, JD Kales, RM Sly, MB Scharf, TL Tan, and TA Preston (1970e): Sleep patterns of asthmatic children: all-night electroencephalographic studies. *J Allergy, 46*:300-308.

Kales, A, EJ Malmstrom, HK Kee, JD Kales, and TL Tan (1969): Effects of hypnotics on sleep patterns, dreaming, and mood state: laboratory and home studies. *Biol Psychiat, 1*:235-241.

Kales, A, TA Preston, TL Tan, and C Allen (1970f): Hypnotics and altered sleep-dream patterns I: all-night EEG studies of glutethimide, methyprylon, and pentobarbital. *Arch Gen Psychiat, 23*:211-218.

Kales, A, TL Tan, EJ Kollar, P Naitoh, TA Preston, and EJ Malmstrom (1970g): Sleep patterns following 205 hours of sleep deprivation. *Psychosom Med, 32*:189-200.

Kales, JD, TL Tan, C Swearingen, and A Kales (1971): Are over-the-counter sleep medications effective? All-night EEG studies. *Curr Therap Res, 13*:143-151.

Kamman, GR (1929): Narcolepsy following epidemic encephalitis. *J Amer Med Assoc, 93*:29-30.

Kane, FJ Jr (1970): Current use of hypnotic drugs: is it rational? *Southern Med J, 63*:376-380.

Karacan, I (1970): Clinical value of nocturnal erection in the prognosis and diagnosis of impotence. *Med Aspects Human Sexuality, 4*:27-34 (April).

Karacan, I, DR Goodenough, A Shapiro, and S Starker (1966a): Erection cycle during sleep in relation to dream anxiety. *Arch Gen Psychiat, 15*:183-189.

Karacan, I, W Heine, HW Agnew Jr, RL Williams, W Webb, and JJ Ross (1968a): Characteristics of sleep patterns during late pregnancy and the postpartum period. *Amer J Obst Gynec, 101*:579-586.

Karacan, I, AL Rosenblum, and RL Williams (1970a): The clitoral erection cycle during sleep (abstract). *Psychophysiol, 7*:338.

Karacan, I, AL Rosenblum, RL Williams, WW Finley, and CJ Hursch (1971): Slow wave sleep deprivation in relation to plasma growth hormone concentration. *Behav Neuropsychiat, 2*:11-14.

Karacan, I, L Schneck, LP Hinterbuchner, and K Gross (1966b): The sleep-dream pattern in Tay-Sachs disease (preliminary observations), from *Inborn Disorders of Sphingolipid Metabolism,* New York, Pergamon, pp. 413-421.

Karacan, I, RL Williams, WW Finley, and CJ Hursch (1970b): The effects of naps on nocturnal sleep: Influence on the need for stage 1-REM and stage 4 sleep. *Biol Psychiat, 2*:391-399.

Karacan, I, RL Williams, CJ Hursch, M McCaulley, and MW Heine (1969a): Some implications of the sleep patterns of pregnancy for postpartum emotional disturbances. *Brit J Psychiat, 115*:929-935.

Karacan, I, RL Williams, and WJ Taylor (1969b): Sleep characteristics of patients with angina pectoris. *Psychosomatics, 10*:280-284.

Karacan, I, SM Wolff, RL Williams, CJ Hursch, and WB Webb (1968b): The effects of fever on sleep and dream patterns. *Psychosomatics, 9*:331-339.

Karadzic, V, and B Mrsulja (1969): Deprivation of paradoxical sleep and brain glycogen. *J Neurochem, 16*:29-34.

Kasamatsu, T (1970): Maintained and evoked unit activity in the mesencephalic reticular formation of the freely behaving cat. *Exp Neurol, 28*: 450-470.

Kasamatsu, A, and T Hirai (1966): An electroencephalograph study on the zen meditation (zazen). *Folia Psychiat Neurol Japon, 20*:315-336.

Kay, DC, RS Eisenstein, and DR Jasinski (1969): Morphine effects on human REM state, waking state and NREM sleep. *Psychopharmacol, 14*:404-416.

Keefe, EB, LC Johnson, and EJ Hunter (1971): EEG and autonomic response pattern during waking and sleep stages. *Psychophysiol, 8*:198-212.

Kennard, MA (1943): Effects on EEG of chronic lesions of basal ganglia, thalamus, and hypothalamus of monkeys. *J Neurophysiol, 6*:405-415.

Kety, SS, EV Evarts, and HL Williams, editors (1967): *Sleep and Altered States of Consciousness.* Baltimore, Williams and Wilkins.

Khazan, N, and CH Sawyer (1964): Mechanisms of paradoxical sleep as revealed by neurophysiologic and pharmacologic approaches in the rabbit. *Psychopharmacol, 5*:457-466.

Kikuchi, S (1969): An electroencephalographic study of nocturnal sleep in temporal lobe epilepsy. *Folia Psychiat Neurol Japon, 23*:59-81.

Kim, C, H Choi, JK Kim, MS Kim, MK Huh, and YB Moon (1971): Sleep pattern of hippocampectomized cat. *Brain Res, 29*:223-236.

King, FA, and PL Marchiafava (1963): Ocular movements in the midpontine pretrigeminal preparation. *Arch Ital Biol, 101*:149-169.

Kleitman, N (1963): *Sleep and Wakefulness,* 2nd ed. Chicago, University of Chicago Press.

Kleitman, N (1969): Basic rest activity cycle in relation to sleep and wakefulness. In A Kales (editor): *Sleep: Physiology and Pathology*. Philadelphia, Lippincott, pp. 33-38.

Klemm, WR (1970): Correlation of hippocampal theta rhythm, movements and brain stem reticular formation activity. *Commun Behav Biol, 5:*147-151.

Knowles, JB, SG Laverty, and HA Kuechler (1968): Effects of alcohol on REM sleep. *Quart J Stud Alc, 29:*342-349.

Koella, WP (1967): *Sleep: Its Nature and Physiological Organization*. Springfield, Thomas.

Koella, WP (1969): Neurohumoral aspects of sleep control. *Biol Psychiat, 1:* 161-177.

Koella, WP (1972): Neurochemical mechanisms of sleep. In Olga Petre-Quadens (editor): *Basic Sleep Mechanisms,* in press.

Koestler, A (1941): *Darkness at Noon*. New York, Macmillan p. 213.

Koestler, A (1967): *The Ghost in the Machine*. New York, Macmillan.

Kollar, EJ, N Namerow, RO Pasnau, and P Naitoh (1968): Neurological findings during prolonged sleep deprivation. *Neurol, 18:*836-840.

Kollar, EJ, RO Pasnau, RT Rubin, P Naitoh, GG Slater, and A Kales (1969): Psychologic, psychophysiologic, and biochemical correlates of prolonged sleep deprivation. *Amer J Psychiat, 126:*488-497.

Komisaruk, BR (1970): Synchrony between limbic system theta activity and rhythmical behavior in rats. *J Comp Physiol Psychol, 70:*482-492.

Kooi, KA (1971): *Fundamentals of Electroencephalography*. New York, Harper and Row, pp. 41-42.

Korner, AF (1968): REM organization in neonates; theoretical implications for development and the biological function of REM. *Arch Gen Psychiat, 19:*330-340.

Kostowski, W, E Giacalone, S Garrattini, and L Valzelli (1968): Studies on behavioural and biochemical changes in rats after lesions of midbrain raphe. *Europ J Pharmacol, 4:*371-376.

Kostowski, W, E Giacalone, S Garrattini, and L Valzelli (1969): Electrical stimulation of midbrain raphe: biochemical, behavioural and bioelectrical effects. *Europ J Pharmacol, 7:*170-175.

Koulack, D (1969): Effects of somatosensory stimulation on dream content. *Arch Gen Psychiat, 20:*718-725.

Koulack, D (1970): Effects of thirst on the sleep cycle. *J Nerv Ment Dis, 151:*143-145.

Kramer, M editor, (1969): *Dream Psychology and the New Biology of Dreaming*. Springfield, Thomas.

Kramer, M, RM Whitman, BJ Baldridge, and LM Lansky (1964): Patterns of dreaming: The interrelationships of the dreams of a night. *J Nerv Ment Dis, 139:*426-439.

Kripke, DF, ML Reite, GV Pegram, LM Stephens, and OF Lewis (1968): Nocturnal sleep in rhesus monkeys. *Electroenceph Clin Neurophysiol, 24:* 582-586.

Kripke, DF, ED Weitzman, and C Pollak (1966): Attempts to induce the rapid eye movement stage of sleep in *Macaca mulatta* by brain stem stimulation. *Psychophysiol, 2:*132-140.

Kuhn, E, V Brodan, M Brodanova, and B Friedmann (1967): Influence of sleep deprivation on iron metabolism. *Nature, 213:*1041-1042.

Kupfer, DJ, HY Meltzer, RJ Wyatt, and F Snyder (1970a): Serum enzyme changes during sleep deprivation. *Nature, 228:*768-769.

Kupfer, DJ, RJ Wyatt, K Greenspond, and F Snyder (1970b): Lithium carbonate and sleep in affective illness. *Arch Gen Psychiat, 23:*35-40.

Kupfer, DJ, RJ Wyatt, J Scott, and F Snyder (1970c): Sleep disturbance in acute schizophrenic patients. *Amer J Psychiat, 126:*1213-1223.

Kupfer, DJ, RJ Wyatt, F Snyder, and JM Davis (1971): Chlorpromazine and sleep in psychiatric patients. *Arch Gen Psychiat, 24:*185-189.

Lamarre, Y, M Filion, and JP Cordeau (1971): Neuronal discharges of the ventrolateral nucleus of the thalamus during sleep and wakefulness in the cat. I. Spontaneous activity. *Exp Brain Res, 12:*480-498.

Larsen, LE, and DO Walter (1970): On automatic methods of sleep staging by EEG spectra. *Electroenceph Clin Neurophysiol, 28:*459-467.

Larson, JD, and WD Foulkes (1969): Electromyogram suppression during sleep, dream recall, and orientation time. *Psychophysiol, 5:*548-555.

Leconte, P, and V Bloch (1970): Deficit de la retention d'un conditionnement apres privation de sommeil paradoxal chez le rat. *Comp Rend Acad Sci, 271:*226-229.

Lehmann, HE (1969): An existential view. In Kramer, M (editor): *Dream Psychology and the New Biology of Dreaming.* Springfield, Thomas, pp. 141-164.

Lenard, HG (1970): The development of sleep spindles in the EEG during the first two years of life. *Neuropediatrie, 1:*264-276.

Lenard, HG, and H Pennigstorff (1970): Alterations in the sleep patterns of infants and young children following acute head injuries. *Acta Pediat Scand, 59:*565-571.

Lenard HG, H von Bermuth, and HFR Prechtl (1968): Reflexes and their relationship to behavioural state in the newborn. *Acta Pediat Scand, 57:* 177-185.

Lessard, CS, and RC Paschall Jr (1970): A system for quantifying EEG slow wave activity. *Electroenceph Clin Neurophysiol, 29:*516-520.

Lesse, H, RG Heath, WA Mickle, RR Monroe, and WH Miller (1955): Rhinencephalic activity during thought. *J Nerv Ment Dis, 122:*433-440.

Lester, BK, JD Coulter, LC Cowden, and HL Williams (1968): Secobarbital and nocturnal physiological patterns. *Psychopharmacol, 13:*275-286.

Lester, BK, JD Coulter, LC Cowden, and HL Williams (1971): Chlorpromazine and human sleep. *Psychopharmacol, 20:*280-287.

Lester, BK, and R Guerrero-Figueroa (1966): Effects of some drugs on electroencephalographic fast activity and dream time. *Psychophysiol, 2:*224-236.

Lewis, SA (1970): Comparative effects of some amphetamine derivatives on human sleep. In E Costa and S Garattini (editors): *Amphetamines and Related Compounds*. New York, Raven, pp. 873-888.

Lewis, SA, and Evans, JI (1969): Dose effects of chlorpromazine on human sleep. *Psychopharmacol, 14*:342-348.

Lewis, SA, I Oswald, JI Evans, MO Akindele, and SL Tompsett (1970): Heroin and human sleep. *Electroenceph Clin Neurophysiol, 28*:374-381.

Levin, M (1936): Periodic somnolence and morbid hunger: a new syndrome. *Brain, 49*:494-504.

Lincoln, DW (1969): Correlation of unit activity in the hypothalamus with EEG patterns associated with the sleep cycle. *Exp Neurol, 24*:1-18.

Lindsley, DB, LH Schreiner, WB Knowles, and HW Magoun (1950): Behavioral and EEG changes following chronic brain stem lesions in the cat. *Electroenceph Clin Neurophysiol, 2*:483-498.

Lorens, SA Jr, and CW Darrow (1962): Eye movements, EEG, GSR and EKG during mental multiplication. *Electroenceph Clin Neurophysiol, 14*: 739-746.

Lowry, FH, JM Cleghorn, and DJ McClure (1971): Sleep patterns in depression: longitudinal study of six patients and brief review of literature. *J Nerv Ment Dis, 153*:10-26.

Lubin, A (1967): Performance under sleep loss and fatigue. In SS Kety, EV Evarts, and HL Williams (editors): *Sleep and Altered States of Consciousness*. Baltimore, Williams and Wilkins, pp. 506-513.

Luce, GG, and J Segal (1966): *Sleep*. New York, Coward-McCann.

Lyman, HM (1885): *Insomnia and Other Disorders of Sleep*. Chicago, Keener.

MacLean, PD (1958): Contrasting functions of limbic and neocortical systems of the brain and their relevance to psychophysiological aspects of medicine. *Amer J Med, 25*:611-626.

MacLean, PD, T Yokota, and MA Kinnard (1968): Photically sustained on-responses of units in posterior hippocampal gyrus of awake monkey. *J Neurophysiol, 31*:870-883.

Madow, L, and LH Snow (1970): *The Psychodynamic Implications of the Physiological Studies on Dreams*. Springfield, Thomas.

Maffei, L, G Moruzzi, and G Rizzolatti (1965): Influence of sleep and wakefulness on the response of lateral geniculate units to sinewave photic stimulation. *Arch Ital Biol, 103*:596-608.

Magnes, J, G Moruzzi, and O Pompeiano (1961): Synchronization of the EEG produced by low-frequency electrical stimulation of the region of the solitary tract. *Arch Ital Biol, 99*:33-67.

Magoun, HW (1954): The ascending reticular system and wakefulness. In JF Delafresnaye (editor): *Brain Mechanisms and Consciousness*. Springfield, Thomas, pp. 1-15.

Magoun, HW (1963): *The Waking Brain*, 2nd ed. Springfield, Thomas.

Malcolm, LJ, JA Watson, and W Burke (1970): PGO waves as unitary events. *Brain Res, 24*:130-133.

Mandell, AJ, B Chaffey, P Brill, MP Mandell, J Rodnick, RT Rubin, and R Sheff (1966): Dreaming sleep in man: changes in urine volume and osmolality. *Science, 151:*1558-1560.

Mandell, AJ, and CE Spooner (1968): Psychochemical research studies in man. *Science, 162:*1442-1453.

Mandell, AJ, CE Spooner, and D Brunet (1969): Whither the "sleep transmitter"? *Biol Psychiat, 1:*13-30.

Mangold, R, L Sokoloff, E Conner, J Kleinerman, PG Therman, and SS Kety (1955): The effects of sleep and lack of sleep on the cerebral circulation and metabolism of normal young men. *J Clin Invest, 34:*1092-1100.

Mano, NI (1970): Changes of simple and complex spike activity of cerebellar Purkinje cells with sleep and waking. *Science, 170:*1325-1327.

Manohar, S, H Noda, and WR Adey (1972): Behavior of mesencephalic reticular neurons in sleep and wakefulness. *Exp Neurol, 34:*140-157.

Marchesi, GF, and P Strata (1970): Climbing fibers of cat cerebellum: modulation of activity during sleep. *Brain Res, 17:*145-148.

Mark, J, L Heiner, P Mandel, and Y Godin (1969): Norepinephrine turnover in brain and stress reactions in rats during paradoxical sleep deprivation. *Life Sci, 8:*1085-1093.

Markham, CH, RD Walter, and LF Chapman (1972): Subcortical sleep activity in man. In PH Crandall and RD Walter (editors): *Epilepsy Originating in the Limbic System.* Cambridge, Harvard University Press, in press.

Marshall, SLA (1962): *Night Drop: The American Airborne Invasion of Normandy.* Boston, Little, Brown.

Mason-Browne, NL (1956): Alteration of consciousness: tumor of the reticular activating system. *Arch Neurol Psychiat, 76:*380-387.

Mattson, RH, KL Pratt, and JR Calverley (1965): Electroencephalograms of epileptics following sleep deprivation. *Arch Neurol, 13:*310-315.

Mazzuchelli-O'Flaherty, AL, JJ O'Flaherty, and R Hernandez Peon (1967): Sleep and other behavioural responses by acetylcholinic stimulation of frontal and mesial cortex. *Brain Res, 4:*268-283.

McCarley, RW, and JA Hobson (1970): Cortical unit activity in desynchronized sleep. *Science, 167:*901-903.

McCrary, JA, and JL Smith (1967): Cortical dyschromatopsia in narcolepsy. *Amer J Ophthal, 64:*153-155.

McGinty, DJ (1969): Somnolence, recovery, and hyposomnia following ventromedial diencephalic lesions in the rat. *Electroenceph Clin Neurophysiol, 26:*70-79.

McGinty, DJ, and MB Sterman (1968): Sleep suppression after basal forebrain lesions in the cat. *Science, 160:*1253-1255.

McNew, JJ, RC Howe, and WR Adey (1971): The sleep cycle and subcortical-cortical relations in the unrestrained chimpanzee. *Electroenceph Clin Neurophysiol, 30:*489-503.

Mellinger, GD, MB Balter, and DI Manheimer (1971): Patterns of psycho-therapeutic drug use among adults in San Francisco. *Arch Gen Psychiat,* 25:385-394.

Mello, NK, and JH Mendelson (1970): Behavioral studies of sleep patterns in alcoholics during intoxication and withdrawal. *J Pharmacol Exp Therap,* 175:94-112.

Mendels, J, and DR Hawkins (1967): Sleep laboratory adaption in normal subjects and depressed patients ("the first night effect"). *Electroenceph Clin Neurophysiol, 22:*556-558.

Mendels, J, and DR Hawkins (1967): Sleep and depression: a controlled EEG study. *Arch Gen Psychiat, 16:*344-354.

Mendels, J, and DR Hawkins (1967): Sleep and depression: a follow-up study. *Arch Gen Psychiat, 16:*536-542.

Mendels, J, and DR Hawkins (1968): Sleep and depression: further considerations. *Arch Gen Psychiat, 19:*445-452.

Mendels, J, and DR Hawkins (1970): Electroencephalographic sleep studies in depression. *Science and Psychoanalysis, 17:*29-46.

Metcalf, DR (1970): EEG sleep spindle ontogenesis. *Neuropadiatrie, 1:*428-433.

Metcalf, DR (1971): Some critical points in normal EEG ontogenesis (abstract). *Electroenceph Clin Neurophysiol, 30:*163.

Micic, D, V Karadzic, and LM Rakic (1967): Changes of gamma-aminobu-tyric acid, glutamic acid, and aspartic acid in various brain structures of cats deprived of paradoxical sleep. *Nature, 215:*169-170.

Miller, JB (1969): Dreams during varying stages of depression. *Arch Gen Psychiat, 20:*560-565.

Mink, WD, PJ Best, and J Olds (1967): Neurons in paradoxical sleep and motivated behavior. *Science, 158:*1335-1337.

Modell, W (1969): Book review. *Clin Pharmacol Therap, 10:*125-126.

Molinari, S, and D Foulkes (1969): Tonic and phasic events during sleep: psychological correlates and implications. *Percept Motor Skills, 29:*343-368.

Monnier, M, T Koller, and S Graber (1963): Humoral influences of induced sleep and arousal upon electrical brain activity of animals with crossed circulation. *Exp Neurol, 8:*264-277.

Monroe, LJ (1967): Psychological and physiological differences between good and poor sleepers. *J Abn Psychol, 72:*255-264.

Monroe, LJ (1969): Inter-rater reliability and the role of experience in scoring EEG sleep records: phase I. *Psychophysiol, 5:*376-384.

Monti (1970): Effect of recurrent stimulation of the brain stem reticular formation on REM sleep in cats. *Exp Neurol, 28:*484-493.

Morden, B, G Mitchell, and WC Dement (1967): Selective REM sleep deprivation and compensation phenomena in the rat. *Brain Res, 5:*339-349.

Morris, GO, HL Williams, and A Lubin (1960): Misperception and disorientation during sleep deprivation. *Arch Gen Psychiat, 2:*247-254.

Morrison, AR, and O Pompeiano (1965): Pyramidal discharge from soma-tosensory cortex and cortical control of primary afferents during sleep. *Arch Ital Biol, 103*:538-568.

Moruzzi, G (1964): Reticular influences on the EEG. *Electroenceph Clin Neurophysiol, 16*:2-17.

Moruzzi, G, and HW Magoun (1949): Brain stem reticular formation and activation of the electroencephalogram. *Electroenceph Clin Neurophysiol, 1*:455-473.

Moskowitz, E, and RJ Berger (1969): Rapid eye movements and dream imagery: are they related? *Nature, 224*:613-614.

Mouret, J, P Bobillier, and M Jouvet (1967): Effets de la parachlorpenylala-nine sur le sommeil du rat. *Comp Rend Soc Biol, 161*:1600-1603.

Mrosovsky, N (1971): *Hibernation and Hypothalamus*. New York, Appleton-Century-Crofts.

Mrsulja, BB, and LM Rakic (1970): The influence of adrenergic and cho-linergic blocking drugs on the glycogen content of the brain in rats deprived of paradoxical sleep. *J Neurochem, 17*:455-456.

Mukhametov, L, and G Rizzolatti (1969): Effect of sleep and waking on flash evoked discharges of lateral geniculate units in unrestrained cats. *Brain Research, 13*:404-406.

Mukhametov, LM, G Rizzolatti, and A Seitun (1970): An analysis of the spontaneous activity of lateral geniculate neurons and of optic tract fibers in free moving cats. *Arch Ital Biol, 108*:325-347.

Mukhametov, LM, G Rizzolatti, and V Tradardi (1970): Spontaneous activity of neurons of nucleus reticularis thalami in freely moving cats. *J Physiol (London), 210*:651-667.

Munson, JB, and RB Graham (1971): Lateral geniculate spikes in sleeping, awake, and reserpine-treated cats: correlated excitability changes in superior colliculus and related structures. *Exp Neurol, 31*:326-336.

Murray, EJ (1965): *Sleep, Dreams, and Arousal*. New York, Appleton-Century-Crofts.

Muzio, JN, HP Roffwarg, and E Kaufman (1966): Alterations in the noc-turnal sleep cycle resulting from LSD. *Electroenceph Clin Neurophysiol, 21*:313-324.

Naitoh, P, LC Johnson, and M Austin (1970): Aquanaut sleep patterns during Tektite I: a 60-day habituation under hyperbaric nitrogen saturation. *Aerospace Med, 42*:69-77.

Nakagawa, Y (1965): Studies on evoked potentials to click and somatosen-sory stimulation in the waking state and during sleep in man. *Folia Psychiat Neurol Japon, 19*:279-293.

Nakamura, Y, and C Ohye (1964): Delta wave production in neocortical EEG by acute lesions within thalamus and hypothalamus of the cat. *Electro-enceph Clin Neurophysiol, 17*:677-684.

Nan'no H, Y Hishikawa, H Koida, H Takahashi, and Z Kaneko (1970): A neurophysiological study of sleep paralysis in narcoleptic patients. *Electroenceph Clin Neurophysiol, 28:*382-390.

Nareloski, J, J Tymicz, and W Lewosz (1969): The circadian sleep of rabbits. *Acta Biol Exp, 29:*185-200.

Natani, K, JT Shurley, CM Pierce, and RE Brooks (1970): Long term changes in sleep patterns in men on the South Polar Plateau. *Arch Intern Med, 125:* 655-659.

Nauta, WJH (1946): Hypothalamic regulation of sleep in rats: an experimental study. *J Neurophysiol, 9:*285-316.

Nauta, WJH (1958): Hippocampal projections and related neural pathways to the midbrain in the cat. *Brain, 81:*319-340.

Nicolis, FB, and Silvestri, LG (1967): Hypnotic activity of placebo in relation to severity of insomnia: a quantitative evaluation. *Clin Pharmacol Therap, 8:*841-848.

Noda, H, S Manohar, and WR Adey (1969): Spontaneous activity of cat hippocampal neurons in sleep and wakefulness. *Exp Neurol, 24:*217-231.

Noda, H, and WR Adey (1970): Changes in neuronal activity in association cortex of the cat in relation to sleep and wakefulness. *Brain Res, 19:*263-275.

Offenkrantz, W, and EA Wolpert (1963): The detection of dreaming in a congenitally blind subject. *J Nerv Ment Dis, 136:*88-90.

Okuma, T, K Nakamura, A Hayaski, and M Fujimori (1966): Psychophysiological study on the depth of sleep in normal human subjects. *Electroenceph Clin Neurophysiol, 21:*140-147.

Olds, J (1962): Hypothalamic substrates of reward. *Physiol Rev, 42:*554-604.

Onheiber, P, PT White, MK DeMyer, and DR Ottinger (1965): Sleep and dream patterns of child schizophrenics. *Arch Gen Psychiat, 12:*568-571.

Oomura, Y, H Ooyama, F Naka, T Yamamoto, T Ono, and N Kobayaski (1969): Some stochastical patterns of single unit discharges in the cat hypothalamus under chronic conditions. *Ann NY Acad Sci, 157:*666-689.

Ornitz, EM, ER Ritvo, MB Brown, S La Franchi, T Parmelee, and RD Walter (1969): The EEG and rapid eye movements during rem sleep in normal and autistic children. *Electroenceph Clin Neurophysiol, 26:*167-175.

Orr, WF, JE Dozier, L Green, and RL Cromwell (1968): Self induced waking: changes in sleep and dream patterns. *Comprehen Psychiat, 9:*499-506.

Orwell, G (1952): *Such, Such Were the Joys.* New York, Harcourt, Brace, p. 16.

Oswald, I (1962): *Sleeping and Waking.* New York, Elsevier.

Oswald, I (1968): Drugs and sleep. *Pharmacol Rev, 20:*272-303.

Oswald, I (1969): Sleep and its disorders. In PJ Vinken and GW Bruyn (editors): *Handbook of Clinical Neurology, Volume 3: Disorders of Higher Nervous Activity.* New York, Wiley, pp. 80-111.

Oswald, I, GW Ashcroft, RJ Berger, D Eccleston, JI Evans, and VR Thacore (1966): Some experiments in the chemistry of normal sleep. *Brit J Psychiat, 112:*391-399.

Oswald, I, RJ Berger, RA Jaramillo, KMG Keddie, PC Olley, and GB Plunkett (1963): Melancholia and barbiturates: a controlled EEG, body, and eye movement study of sleep. *Brit J Psychiat, 109:*66-78.

Oswald, I, HS Jones, and JE Mannerheim (1968): Effects of two slimming drugs on sleep. *Brit Med J, 1:*796-799.

Oswald, I, and RG Priest (1965): Five weeks to escape the sleeping pill habit. *Brit Med J, 2:*1093-1099.

Oswald, I, AM Taylor, and M Treisman (1960): Discriminative responses to stimulation during human sleep. *Brain, 83:*440-453.

Oswald, I, and VR Thacore (1963): Amphetamine and phenmetrazine addiction: physiological abnormalities in the abstinence syndrome. *Brit Med J, 2:*427-431.

Othmer, E, DR Goodwin, WR Levine, JA Halikas, and FR Freemon (1970): Short latency REM in alcoholics (abstract), *Psychophysiol, 7:*347.

Othmer, E, MP Hayden, and R Segelbaum (1969): Encephalic cycles during sleep and wakefulness in humans: a 24 hour pattern. *Science, 164:*447-449.

Owen, M, and EL Bliss (1970): Sleep loss and cerebral excitability. *Amer J Physiol, 218:*171-173.

Parker, DC, and LG Rossman (1971): Human growth hormone release in sleep: nonsuppression by acute hyperglycemia. *J Clin Endocrinol Metab, 32:*65-69.

Parker, DC, JF Sassin, JW Mace, RW Gotlin, and LG Rossman (1969): Human growth hormone release during sleep: electroencephalographic correlation. *J Clin Endocrinol Metab, 29:*871-874.

Parker, HL (1956): *Clinical Studies in Neurology.* Springfield, Thomas, pp. 231-238.

Parmalee, AH, Y Akiyama, E Stern, and MA Harris (1969): A periodic cerebral rhythm in newborn infants. *Exp Neurol, 25:*575-584.

Parmalee, AH, FJ Schulte, Y Akiyama, WH Wenner, MA Schultz, and E Stern (1968): Maturation of EEG activity during sleep in premature infants. *Electroenceph Clin Neurophysiol, 24:*319-329.

Parmeggiani, PL (1962): Sleep behavior elicited by electrical stimulation of cortical and subcortical structures in the cat. *Helv Physiol Acta, 20:*347-367.

Parmeggiani (1967): On the functional significance of the hippocampal theta rhythm. *Prog Brain Res, 27:*413-441.

Parmeggiani, PL, and C Franzini (1970): Activity of hypothalamic units during sleep (abstract). *Experientia, 26:*682.

Parmeggiani, PL, and C Franzini (1971): Changes in the activity of hypothalamic units during sleep at different environmental temperatures. *Brain Res, 29:*347-350.

Parmeggiani, PL, and C Rabini (1970): Sleep and environmental temperature. *Arch Ital Biol, 108:*369-387.

Parmeggiani, PL, and G Zanocco (1963): A study on the bioelectrical rhythms of cortical and subcortical structures during activated sleep. *Arch Ital Biol, 101*:385-412.

Passouant, P, J Cadilhac, M Baldy-Moulinier, and C Mion (1970): Etude du sommeil nocturne chez des uremiques chroniques soumis a une epuration extrarenale. *Electroenceph Clin Neurophysiol, 29*:441-449.

Passouant, P, L Popoviciu, G Velok, and M Baldy-Moulinier (1968): Etude polygraphique des narcolepsies au cours du nycthemere. *Rev Neurol (Paris), 118*:431-441.

Patry, G, S Lyagoubi, and CA Tassinari (1971): Subclinical "electrical status epilepticus" induced by sleep in children. *Arch Neurol, 24*:242-252.

Pauker, SG (1970): Grand-rounds whiplash. *New Engl J Med, 283*:600-601.

Pearlman, CA (1970): The adaptive function of dreaming. *Int Psychiat Clinics, 7*:329-334.

Penaloza-Rojas, JH, M Elterman, and N Olmos (1964): Sleep induced by cortical stimulation. *Exp Neurol, 10*:140-147.

Persson, T, L Olsson, and E Ortmann (1969): The Kleine-Levin syndrome: report of a case and discussion. *Behav Neuropsychiat, 1*:4-6.

Petre-Quadens, O (1966): On the different phases of sleep of the newborn with special reference to the activated phase or phase d. *J Neurol Sci, 3*:151-161.

Petre-Quadens, O (1967): Ontogenesis of paradoxical sleep in the human newborn. *J Neurol Sci, 4*:153-157.

Petre-Quadens, O, editor (1972): *Basic Sleep Mechanisms.* Springfield, Thomas.

Petre-Quadens, O, and C de Lee (1970): Eye movements during sleep: a common criterion of learning capacities and endocrine activity. *Develop Med Child Neurol, 12*:730-740.

Petre-Quadens, O, and M Jouvet (1966): Paradoxical sleep and dreaming in the mentally retarded. *J Neurol Sci, 3*:608-612.

Petre-Quadens, O, and M Jouvet (1967): Sleep in the mentally retarded. *J Neurol Sci, 4*:354-357.

Pfeiffer, JE (1969): *The Emergence of Man.* New York, Harper and Row, pp. 55-56.

Pillard, RC (1970): Marihuana. *New Eng J Med, 283*:294-303.

Pisano, M, G Rosadini, GF Rossi, and J Zattoni (1966): Relations between threshold of arousal and electroencephalographic patterns during sleep in man. *Physiol Behav 1*:55-58.

Pivik, RT, V Zarcone, WC Dement, and LE Hollister (1972): Delta-9 tetrahydrocannabinol and synhexl: effects on human sleep patterns. *Clin Pharmacol Therap, 13*:426-435.

Pivik, T, and WD Foulkes (1968): NREM Mentation: relation to personality, orientation time, and time of night. *J Consult Clin Psychol, 32*:144-151.

Podvoll, EM, and SJ Goodman (1967): Averaged neural electrical activity and arousal. *Science, 155*:223-225.

Pompeiano, O (1969): Sleep mechanisms. In HH Jasper, AA Ward Jr, and A Pope (editors): *Basic Mechanisms of the Epilepsies.* Boston, Little, Brown, pp. 453-473.

Pompeiano, O, and JE Swett (1962): EEG and behavioral manifestations of sleep induced by cutaneous nerve stimulation in normal cats. *Arch Ital Biol, 100:*311-342.

Pompeiano, O, and JE Swett (1962): Identification of cutaneous and muscular afferent fibers producing EEG synchronization or arousal in normal cats. *Arch Ital Biol, 100:*343-373.

Pond, DA (1952): Narcolepsy: a brief critical review and study of eight cases. *J Ment Sci, 98:*595-604.

Pratt, KL, RH Mattson, NJ Weikers, and R Williams (1968): EEG activation of epileptics following sleep deprivation: a prospective study of 114 cases. *Electroenceph Clin Neurophysiol, 24:*11-15.

Prechtl, HFR (1970): Brain and behavioural mechanisms in the human new-born infant. In R Robinson (editor): *Brain and Early Behavior.* New York, Academic, pp. 115-138.

Prechtl, HFR (1972): Sleep in the newborn infant: mathematical analysis of polygraphic recordings and system analysis of sleep. In Olga Petre-Quadens (editor): *Basic Sleep Mechanisms,* in press.

Prechtl, HFR, and HG Lenard (1967): A study of eye movements in sleeping newborn infants. *Brain Research, 5:*477-493.

Prechtl, HFR, V Vlach, HG Lenard, and DK Grant (1967): Exteroceptive and tendon reflexes in various behavioural states in the newborn infant. *Biol Neonat, 11:*159-175.

Pujol, JF, A Buguet, JL Froment, B Jones, and M Jouvet (1971): The central metabolism of serotonin in the cat during insomnia: a neurophysiological and biochemical study after administration of p-chlorophenylalanine or destruction of the raphe system. *Brain Res, 29:*195-212.

Pujol, JF, J Mouret, M Jouvet, and J Glowinski (1968): Increased turnover of cerebral norepinephrine during rebound of paradoxical sleep in the rat. *Science, 159:*112-114.

Purpura, DP (1969): Interneuronal mechanisms in thalamically induced synchronizing and desynchronizing activities. In MAB Brazier (editor): *The Interneuron.* Los Angeles, Univ of Calif Press, pp. 467-496.

Purpura, DP (1972): Intracellular studies of thalamic synaptic mechanisms in evoked synchronization and desynchronization of electrocortical activity. In Olga Petre-Quadens (editor): *Basic Sleep Mechanisms,* in press.

Ranson, SW (1939): Somnolence caused by hypothalamic lesions in the monkey. *Arch Neurol Psychiat, 41:*1-23.

Raybin, JB, and TP Detre (1969): Sleep disorder and symptomatology among medical and nursing students. *Comprehen Psychiat, 10:*452-462.

Rechtschaffen, A, and L Maron (1964): The effect of amphetamine on the sleep cycle. *Electroenceph Clin Neurophysiol, 16:*438-445.

Rechtschaffen, A, and B Roth (1969): Nocturnal sleep of hypersomniacs. *Activitas Nervosa Superior, 11*:229-233.

Rechtschaffen, A, G Vogel, and G Shaikun (1963): Interrelatedness of mental activity during sleep. *Arch Gen Psychiat, 9*:536-547.

Rechtschaffen, A, EA Wolpert, WC Dement, SA Mitchell, and C Fisher (1963): Nocturnal sleep of narcoleptics. *Electroenceph Clin Neurophysiol, 15*:599-609.

Reyher, J, and H Morishige (1969): Electroencephalogram and rapid eye movements during free imagery and dream recall. *J Abn Psychol, 74*:576-582.

Rhodes, JM (1969): Electrical activity of the brain as a reflection of inhibitory phenomena. *Neuropsychologia, 7*:209-216.

Rhodes, JM, WR Adey, RT Kado, and ML Reite (1963): Differing EEG sleep stages and their response to tone stimulation in the chimp. *Physiologist, 6*:264.

Rhodes, JM, CM McGinnis, GV Pegram, and E Balzano (1971): Developmental aspects of the chimpanzee EEG (abstract). *Electroenceph Clin Neurophysiol, 30*:159-165.

Rhodes, JM, ML Reite, D Brown, and WR Adey (1964): Cortical subcortical relationships in the chimpanzee during different phases of sleep (abstract). *Electroencephal Clin Neurophysiol, 17*:449.

Rickles, WR (1965): A study of EEG and somato-vegetative physiology of the immature chimpanzee during sleep. *Aeromedical Res Lab Tech Rept No 64-19.* Holloman Air Force Base, New Mexico.

Ritvo, ER, EM Ornitz, S LaFranchi, and RD Walter (1967): Effects of imipramine on the sleep-dream cycle: an EEG study in boys. *Electroenceph Clin Neurophysiol, 22*:465-468.

Robin, ED (1958): Some interrelations between sleep and disease. *Arch Int Med, 102*:669-675.

Rodden, A, A Sinha, WC Dement, and J Barchas (1970): Altered C14 leucine incorporation into brain protein of sleeping rats (abstract) *Psychophysiol, 7*:312-313.

Roelofs, GA, RH van den Hoofdakker, and HFR Prechtl (1963): Sleep effects of subliminal brain stimulation in cats. *Exp Neurol, 8*:84-92.

Roessler, R, F Collins, and R Ostman (1970): A period analysis classification of sleep stages. *Electroenceph Clin Neurophysiol, 29*:358-362.

Roffwarg, HP, WC Dement, JN Muzio, and C Fisher (1962): Dream imagery: relationship to rapid eye movements of sleep. *Arch Gen Psychiat, 7*:235-258.

Roffwarg, HP, JN Muzio, and WC Dement (1966): Ontogenetic development of the human sleep-dream cycle. *Science, 152*:604-619.

Rojas-Ramirex, JA, and ES Tauber (1970): Paradoxical sleep in two species of avian predator (Falconiformes). *Science, 167*:1754-1755.

Roldan, E, T Weiss, and E Fifkova (1963): Excitability changes during the sleep cycle of the rat. *Electroenceph Clin Neurophysiol, 15*:775-785.

Rosenbloom, AL, I Karacan, and FL DeBusk (1970): Sleep characteristics and endocrine responses in progeria. *J Pediatrics, 77*:692-695.

Ross, JJ (1965): Neurological findings after prolonged sleep deprivation. *Arch Neurol, 12:*399-403.

Ross, JJ, HW Agnew Jr, RL Williams, and WB Webb (1968): Sleep patterns in pre-adolescent children: an EEG-EOG study. *Pediatrics, 42:*324-335.

Ross, JJ, LC Johnson, and RD Walter (1966): Spike and wave discharges during stages of sleep. *Arch Neurol, 14:*399-407.

Roth, B, S Bruhova, and M Lehovsky (1969): REM sleep and NREM sleep in narcolepsy and hypersomnia. *Electroenceph Clin Neurophysiol, 26:*176-182.

Rougeul, A, A LeYaouanc, and P Buser (1966): Activities neuroniques spontanees dans le tractus pyramidal et certaines structures sous-corticales au cours du sommeil naturel chez le chat libre. *Exp Brain Res, 2:*129-150.

Routtenberg, A (1966): Neural mechanisms of sleep: changing view of reticular formation function. *Psychol Rev, 73:*481-499.

Routtenberg, A (1968): The two-arousal hypothesis: reticular formation and limbic system. *Psychol Rev, 75:*51-80.

Rubin, RT, A Kales, R Adler, T Fagan, and W Odell (1972): Gonadotropin secretion during sleep in normal adult men. *Science, 175:*196-198.

Rubin, RT, A Kales, and BR Clark (1969): Decreased 17 hydroxycorticosteroid and VMA excretion during sleep following glutethimide administration in man. *Life Sci, 17:*959-964.

Ruckebusch, Y (1962): Activite corticale au cours du sommeil chez la chevre. *Comp Rend Soc Biol, 156:*691-708.

Ruckebusch, Y (1963): Etude poligraphique et comportementale de l'evolution postnatale du sommeil physiologique chez l'agneau. *Arch Ital Biol, 101:*111-132.

Ruckebusch, Y (1963): Etude EEG et comportementale des alternances veille-sommeil chez l'ane. *Comp Rend Soc Biol, 157:*840-844.

Ruckebush, Y, and J Bost (1962): Activite corticale au cours de la somnolence et de la rumination chez la chevre. *J Physiol, 54:*409-410.

Ruckebusch, Y, and MT Morel (1968): Etude polygraphique du sommeil chez le porc. *Comp Rend Soc Biol, 162:*1346-1354.

Safer, DJ (1970a): The effect of LSD on sleep deprived men. *Psychopharmacol, 17:*414-424.

Safer, DJ (1970b): The concomitant effects of mild sleep loss and an anticholinergic drug. *Psychopharmacol, 17:*425-433.

Sagales, T, S Erill, and EF Domino (1969): Differential effects of scopolamine and chlorpromazine on REM and NREM sleep in normal male subjects. *Clin Pharmacol Therap, 10:*522-529.

Sainsbury, RS (1970): Hippocamal activity during natural behavior in the guinea pig. *Physiol Behav, 5:*317-324.

Sakakura, H (1968): Spontaneous and evoked unitary activities of cat lateral geniculate neurons in sleep and wakefulness. *Jap J Physiol, 18:*23-42.

Salamy, J (1970): Instrumental responding to internal cues associated with REM sleep. *Psychonom Sci, 18:*342-343.

Sampson, H (1965): Deprivation of dreaming sleep by two methods: Compensatory REM time. *Arch Gen Psychiat, 13:*79-86.

Sampson H (1966): Psychological effects of deprivation of dreaming sleep. *J Nerv Ment Dis, 143:*305-317.

Sassin, JF, JH Jacoby, J Finkelstein, D Fukushima, and E Weitzman (1971): Episodic release of growth hormone and cortisol in monkeys (abstract). *Neurol, 21:*431-432.

Sassin, JF, DC Parker, JW Mace, RW Gotlin, LC Johnson, and LG Rossman (1969): Human growth hormone release: relation to slow-wave sleep and sleep-waking cycles. *Science, 165:*513-515.

Schapiro, A (1967): Dreaming and the physiology of sleep: A critical review of some empirical data and a proposal for a theoretical model of sleep and dreaming. *Exp Neurol Suppl, 4:*56-81.

Scheibel, ME, and AB Scheibel (1958): Structural substrates for integrative patterns in the brain stem reticular core. In HH Jasper and LD Proctor (editors): *Reticular Formation of the Brain.* Boston, Little, Brown, pp. 31-55.

Scheibel, ME, and AB Scheibel (1966): The organization of the nucleus reticularis thalami. *Brain Res, 1:*43-62.

Scheibel, ME, and AB Scheibel (1967): Structural organization of nonspecific thalamic nuclei and their projection toward cortex. *Brain Res, 6:*60-94.

Schiff, SK (1965): The EEG, eye movements and dreaming in adult enuresis. *J Nerv Ment Dis, 140:*397-404.

Schmidt, HS, and R Kaelbling (1971): The differential laboratory adaption of sleep parameters. *Biol Psychiat, 3:*33-45.

Schultz, MA, FJ Schulte, Y Akiyama, and AH Parmelee Jr (1968): Development of electroencephalographic sleep phenomena in hypothyroid infants. *Electroenceph Clin Neurophysiol, 25:*351-358.

Schwartz, BA, and C Escande (1970): Sleeping sickness: sleep study of a case. *Electroenceph Clin Neurophysiol, 29:*83-87.

Scollo-Lavizzari, G (1970): A note on cataplexy with simultaneous EEG recordings. *Europ Neurol, 4:*57-63.

Shaywitz, BA, J Finkelstein, L Hellman, and ED Weitzman (1971): Growth hormone in newborn infants during sleep-wake periods. *Pediatrics, 48:*103-109.

Shimazono, Y, T Horie, Y Yanagisawa, N Hori, S Chikazawa, and K Shozuka (1960): The correlation of the rhythmic waves of the hippocampus with the behavior of dogs. *Neurol Med Chir, 2:*82-88.

Siegel, J, and TP Gordon (1965): Paradoxical sleep deprivation in the cat. *Science, 148:*978-980.

Siegel, J, and TD Langley (1965): Arousal threshold in the cat as a function of sleep phase and stimulus significance. *Experientia, 21:*740-741.

Silverman, D, and A Morisaki (1958): A re-evaluation of sleep electroencephalography. *Electroenceph Clin Neurophysiol, 10:*425-431.

Slocombe, G (1959): *William The Conqueror.* New York, Putnam, p. 16.

Slosarska, M, and B Zernicki (1969): Synchronized sleep in the chronic pretrigeminal cat. *Acta Biol Exp, 29:*175-184.

Small, A, S Hibi, and I Feinberg (1971): Effects of dextroamphetamine sulfate on EEG sleep patterns of hyperactive children. *Arch Gen Psychiat, 25:* 369-380.

Smith, CM (1959): Electroencephalogram in cataplexy. *Electroenceph Clin Neurophysiol, 11:*344-345.

Smith, E (1968): *Brief Against Death*. New York, Knopf.

Snyder, F (1966): Toward an evolutionary theory of dreaming. *Amer J Psychiat, 123:*121-136.

Snyder, F (1967): In quest of dreaming. In HA Witkin and HB Lewis (editors): *Experimental Studies of Dreaming*. New York, Random House, pp. 3-75.

Snyder, F (1969): Dynamic aspects of sleep disturbance in relation to mental illness. *Biol Psychiat, 1:*119-130.

Snyder, F, JA Hobson, DF Morrison, and F Goldfrank (1964): Changes in respiration, heart rate, and systolic blood pressure in human sleep. *J Appl Physiol, 19:*417-422.

Solomon, P (1956): Insomnia. *New Engl J Med, 255:*755-760.

Soulairac, A, C Gottesmann, and MJ Thangapregassam (1965): Etude electro-physiologique des differentes phases de sommeil chez le rat. *Arch Ital Biol, 103:*469-482.

Sours, JA (1963): Narcolepsy and other disturbances in the sleep-waking rhythm: a study of 115 cases with review of the literature. *J Nerv Ment Dis, 137:*525-542.

Starr, A (1967): A disorder of rapid eye movements in Huntington's chorea. *Brain, 90:*545-564.

Sterman, MB, and CD Clemente (1962): Forebrain inhibitory mechanisms: sleep patterns induced by basal forebrain stimulation in the behaving cat. *Exp Neurol, 6:*103-117.

Sterman, MB, T Knauss, D Lehmann, and CD Clemente (1965): Circadian sleep and waking patterns in the laboratory cat. *Electroenceph Clin Neuro-physiol, 19:*509-517.

Stern, M, DH Fram, R Wyatt, L Grinspoon, and B Tursky (1969): All-night sleep studies of acute schizophrenics. *Arch Gen Psychiat, 20:*470-477.

Stern, M, H Roffwarg, and R Duvoisin (1968): The parkinsonian tremor in sleep. *J Nerv Ment Dis, 147:*202-210.

Stevens, JR, H Kodama, B Lonsbury, and L Mills (1971): Ultradian characteristics of spontaneous seizure discharges recorded by radio telemetry in man. *Electroenceph Clin Neurophysiol, 31:*313-325.

Storms, MD, and RE Nisbett (1970): Insomnia and the attribution process. *J Personality Social Psychol, 16:*319-328.

Stossel, TP (1970): The forgotten aspect of medical education. *Pharos, 33:* 16-18.

Suzuki, J (1966): Narcoleptic syndrome and paradoxical sleep. *Folia Psychiat Neurol Japon, 20:*123-149.

Symonds, C (1954): Cataplexy and other related forms of seizure. *Canad Med Assoc J, 70:*621-625.

Takahashi, Y, DM Kipnis, and WH Daughaday (1968): Growth hormone secretion during sleep. *J Clin Invest, 47:*2079-2090.

Tart, CT (1970): Waking from sleep at a preselected time. *J Amer Soc Psychosom Dent Med, 17:*3-16.

Tauber, ES, J Rojas-Ramirez, and R Hernandez Peon (1968): Electro-physiological and behavioral correlates of wakefulness and sleep in the lizard, *Ctenosaura pectinata. Electroenceph Clin Neurophysiol, 24:*424-433.

Thacore, VR, H Ahmed, and I Oswald (1969): The EEG in a case of periodic hypersomnia. *Electroenceph Clin Neurophysiol, 27:*605-606.

Thomas, EM (1959): *The Harmless People.* New York, Knopf, p. 39.

Timo-Iaria, C, N Negrao, WR Schmidek, K Hoshino, CE Lobato de Menezes, and T Leme da Rocha (1970): Phases and states of sleep in the rat. *Physiol Behav, 5:*1057-1062.

Torda, C (1967): Sleeping and dreaming mechanism. *Lancet, 1:*1011.

Torda, C (1968): Contribution to serotonin theory of dreaming (LSD infusion). *NY State J Med. 68:*1135-1138.

Torda, C (1969): Biochemical and bioelectric processes related to sleep, paradoxical sleep, and arousal. *Psychol Rep, 24:*807-824.

Torda C (1969): Dreams of subjects with bilateral hippocampal lesions. *Acta Psychiat Scand, 45:*277-288.

Toyoda, J (1964): The effects of chlorpromazine and imipramine on the human nocturnal sleep electroencephalogram. *Folia Psychiat Neurol Japon, 18:* 198-221.

Toyoda, J, K Sasaki, and M Kurihara (1966): A polygraphic study on the effect of atropine on human nocturnal sleep. *Folia Psychiat Neurol Japon, 20:*275-289.

Traczyk, WZ, DI Whitmoyer, and CH Sawyer (1969): EEG feedback control of midbrain electrical stimulation inducing sleep or arousal in rabbits. *Acta Biol Exp, 29:*135-152.

Traczynska-Kubin, D, E Atzef, and O Petre-Quadens (1969): Le sommeil dans la maladie de Parkinson. *Acta Neurol Psychiat Belg, 69:*727-733.

Trosman, H (1963): Dream research and the psychoanalytic theory of dreams. *Arch Gen Psychiat, 9:*9-18.

Tsuchiya, K, M Toru, and T Kobayaski (1969): Sleep deprivation: changes of monoamines and acetylcholine in rat brain. *Life Sci, 8:*867-873.

Tune, GS (1968): Sleep and wakefulness in normal human adults. *Brit Med J 2:*269-271.

Tune, GS (1969): Sleep and wakefulness in 509 normal human adults. *Brit J Med Psychol, 42:*75-80

Ullman, M (1958): Dreams and arousal. *Amer J Psychother, 12:*222-233.

Ullman, M, and S Krippner (1970): *Dream Studies and Telepathy: An Experimental Approach.* New York, Parapsychology Foundation.

Ursin, R (1968): The 2 stages of slow-wave sleep in the cat and their relation to REM sleep. *Brain Res, 11:*347-356.

Valleala, P (1967): The temporal relation of unit discharge in visual cortex and activity of the extraocular muscles during sleep. *Arch Ital Biol, 105:* 1-14.

Van den Noort, S, and K Brine (1970): Effect of sleep on brain labile phosphates and metabolic rate. *Amer J Physiol, 218:*1434-1439.

Vanderwolf, CH (1969): Hippocampal electrical activity and voluntary movement in the rat. *Electroenceph Clin Neurophysiol, 26:*407-418.

Vasilescu, E (1970): Sleep and wakefulness in the tortise *(Emys orbicularis). Rev Roum Biol Zool, 15:*177-179.

Velluti, R, and R Hernandez-Peon (1963): Atropine blockade within a cholinergic hypnogenic circuit. *Exp Neurol, 8:*20-29.

Verdone, P (1965): Temporal reference of manifest dream content. *Percept Mot Skills, 20:*1253-1268.

Verdone, P (1968): Sleep satiation: extended sleep in normal subjects. *Electroenceph Clin Neurophysiol, 24:*417-423.

Villablanca, J (1965): The electrocorticogram in the cerveau isole cat. *Electroenceph Clin Neurophysiol, 19:*576-586.

Vincent, JD, O Benoit, J Scherrer, and JM Faure (1967): Activites elementaires recueillies dans l' hypothalamus au cours de la veille et du sommeil chez le Lapin chronique (abstract). *J Physiol (Paris), 59:*527.

Vitale-Neugebauer, A, A Giuditta, B Vitale, and S Giaquinto (1970): Pattern of RNA synthesis in rabbit cortex during sleep. *J Neurochem, 17:*1263-1273.

Vogel, GW (1968): REM deprivation: III. Dreaming and psychosis. *Arch Gen Psychiat, 18:*312-329.

Vogel, G, D Foulkes, and H Trosman (1966): Ego functions and dreaming during sleep onset. *Arch Gen Psychiat, 14:*238-248.

Vogel, GW, and AC Traub (1968): REM deprivation: I. The effect on schizophrenic patients. *Arch Gen Psychiat, 18:*287-300.

Vogel, GW, AC Traub, P Ben-Horin, and GM Meyers (1968): REM deprivation: II. The effects on depressed patients. *Arch Gen Psychiat, 18:*301-311.

Wageneder, FM, and S Schuy, editors (1970): *Electrotherapeutic Sleep and Electroanesthesia.* Excerpta Med.

Watkins, AV (1969): *Enough Rope.* New York, Prentice-Hall, p. 1.

Webb, WB (1968): *Sleep: An Experimental Approach.* New York, Macmillan.

Webb, WB, and JK Friedmann (1971): Some temporal characteristics of paradoxical (LVF) sleep occurrence in the rat. *Electroenceph Clin Neurophysiol, 30:*453-456.

Weiss, B, and VG Laties (1962): Enhancement of human performance by caffeine and amphetamines. *Pharmacol Rev, 14:*1-36.

Weiss, E, B Bordwell, M Seeger, J Lee, WC Dement, and J Barchas (1968): Changes in brain serotonin (5HT) and 5-hydroxyindole 3-acetic acid (5HIAA) in REM sleep deprived rats (abstract). *Psychophysiol, 5:209.*

Weiss, T, and E Roldan (1964): Comparative study of sleep cycles in rodents. *Experientia, 20:280-281.*

Weisz, R, and D Foulkes (1970): Home and laboratory dreams collected under uniform sampling conditions. *Psychophysiol, 6:588-596.*

Weitzman, ED, and H Kremen (1965): Auditory evoked responses during different stages of sleep in man. *Electroenceph Clin Neurophysiol, 18:65-70.*

Weitzman, ED, DF Kripke, C Pollak, and J Dominguez (1965): Cyclic activity in sleep of *Macaca mulatta. Arch Neurol, 12:463-467.*

Weitzman, ED, MM Rapport, and JJ McGregor (1968): Sleep patterns of the monkey and brain serotonin concentration: effect of p-chlorphenylalanine. *Science, 160:1361-1363.*

West, LJ (1969): Introduction: the dream in behavioral science. In M Kramer (editor): *Dream Psychology and the New Biology of Dreaming,* Springfield, Thomas, pp. xvi-xxiv.

Whitehead, WE, TM Robinson, MZ Wincor, and A Rechtschaffen (1969): The accumulation of REM sleep need during sleep and wakefulness. *Comm Behav Biol, 4:195-201.*

Whitfield, IC (1968): Centrifugal control mechanisms of the auditory pathway. In Ciba Foundation Symposium, *Hearing Mechanisms in Vertebrates.* London, Churchill, pp. 246-254.

Whitlock, DG, A Arduini, and G Moruzzi (1953): Microelectrode analysis of pyramidal system during transition from sleep to wakefulness. *J Neurophysiol, 16:414-429.*

WHO Expert Committee on Drug Dependence (1969): Sixteenth report. *WHO Techn Rep Ser, 407:5-28.*

Wilkinson, RT (1968): Sleep deprivation: performance tests for partial and selective sleep deprivation. *Prog Clin Psychol, 8:28-43.*

Williams, DH, and RD Cartwright (1969): Blood pressure changes during EEG-monitored sleep. *Arch Gen Psychiat, 20:307-314.*

Williams, HL, JT Hammack, RL Daly, WC Dement, and A Lubin (1964): Responses to auditory stimulation, sleep loss and the EEG stages of sleep. *Electroenceph Clin Neurophysiol, 16:269-279.*

Williams, HL, Lester, BK, and Coulter, JD (1969a): Monoamines and the EEG stages of sleep. *Activitas Nervosa Superior, 11:188-192.*

Williams, HL, BK Lester, and JD Coulter (1969b): Alpha chloralose and nocturnal physiological patterns. *Psychopharmacol, 15:28-38.*

Williams, HL, HC Morlock Jr, and JV Morlock (1966): Instrumental behavior during sleep. *Psychophysiol, 2:208-216.*

Williams, HL, DI Tepas, and HC Morlock Jr (1962): Evoked responses to clicks and electroencephalographic stages of sleep in man. *Science, 138:685-686.*

Williams, RL and Agnew, HW, Jr (1969): The effects of drugs on the EEG sleep patterns of normal humans. *Exp Med Surg, 27*:53-64.

Williams, RL, HW Agnew Jr, and WB Webb (1964): Sleep patterns in young adults: an EEG study. *Electroenceph Clin Neurophysiol, 17*:376-381.

Williams, RL, HW Agnew Jr, and WB Webb (1966): Sleep patterns in young females: an EEG study. *Electroenceph Clin Neurophysiol, 20*:264-266.

Williams, RL and WB Webb (1966): *Sleep Therapy: A Bibliography and Commentary.* Springfield, Thomas.

Wilson, SAK (1928): The narcolepsies. *Brain, 51*:63-109.

Wilson, WP, and BS Nashold (1969): The sleep rhythms of subcortical nuclei: some observations in man. *Biol Psychiat, 1*:289-296.

Wilson, WP, and WWK Zung (1966): Attention, discrimination, and arousal during sleep. *Arch Gen Psychiat, 15*:523-528

Winokur, G, and T Reich (1970): Two genetic factors in manic-depressive disease. *Comprehen Psychiat, 11*:93-99.

Winters, WD, K Mori, CE Spooner, and RT Kado (1967): Correlation of reticular and cochlear multiple unit activity with auditory evoked responses during wakefulness and sleep. *Electroenceph Clin Neurophysiol, 23*:539-545.

Witkin, HA, and HB Lewis, editors (1967): *Experimental Studies of Dreaming.* New York, Random.

Wolbarsht, ML, EF MacNichol Jr, and HG Wagner (1960): Glass insulated platinum microelectrode. *Science, 132*:1309-1310.

Wolpert, EA (1960): Studies in psychophysiology of dreams II: an electro-myographic study of dreaming. *Arch Gen Psychiat, 2*:231-241.

Wolpert, EA (1968): Psychophysiologic parallelism in the dream. *Prog Clin Psychol, 8*:76-90.

Wulfsohn, NL, and A Sances Jr, editors (1970): *The Nervous System and Electric Currents.* New York, Plenum.

Wyatt, RJ, TN Chase, J Scott, and F Snyder (1970a): Effect of L-dopa on the sleep of man. *Nature, 228*:999-1000.

Wyatt, RJ, K Engleman, DJ Kupfer, DH Fram, A Sjoerdsma, and F Snyder (1970b): Effects of L-tryptophan (a natural sedative) on human sleep. *Lancet, 2*:842-845.

Wyatt, RJ, K Engleman, DJ Kupfer, J Scott, A Sjoerdsma, and F Synder (1969a): Effects of para-chlorophenylalanine on sleep in man. *Electroenceph Clin Neurophysiol, 27*:529-532.

Wyatt, RJ, DH Fram, R Buchbinder, and F Snyder (1971a): Treatment of intractable narcolepsy with a monoamine oxidase inhibitor. *New Engl J Med, 285*:987-991.

Wyatt, RJ, DH Fram, DJ Kupfer, and F Snyder (1971b): Total prolonged drug-induced REM sleep suppression in anxious-depressed patients. *Arch Gen Psychiat, 24*:145-155.

Wyatt, RJ, DJ Kupfer, J Scott, DS Robinson, and F Snyder (1969b): Longitudinal studies of the effect of monoamine oxidase inhibitors on sleep in man. *Psychopharmacol, 15*:236-244.

Wyatt, RJ, V Zarcone, K Engleman, WC Dement, F Snyder, and A Sjoerdsma (1971c): Effects of 5-hydroxytryptophan on the sleep of normal human subjects. *Electroenceph Clin Neurophysiol, 30:*505-509.

Yamamoto, J, E Furuya, H Wakamatsu, and Y Hishikawa (1971): Modification of photosensitivity in epileptics during sleep. *Electroenceph Clin Neurophysiol, 31:*509-513.

Yules, RB, DX Freedman, and K Chandler (1966): The effect of ethyl alcohol on man's electroencephalographic sleep cycle. *Electroenceph Clin Neurophysiol, 20:*109-111.

Yules, RB, ME Lipman, and DX Freedman (1967): Alcohol administration prior to sleep. *Arch Gen Psychiat, 16:*94-97.

Zir, LM, RA Smith, and DC Parker (1971): Human growth hormone release in sleep: effect of daytime exercise. *J Clin Endocrinol Metab, 32:*662-665.

Zung, WWK (1969): Antidepressant drugs and sleep. *Exp Med Surg, 27:* 124-137.

Zung, WWK (1969): Effect of antidepressant drugs on sleeping and dreaming: III on the depressed patient. *Biol Psychiat, 1:*283-287.

Zung, WWK, and WP Wilson (1971): Time estimation during sleep. *Biol Psychiat, 3:*159-164.

Zung, WWK, WP Wilson, and WE Dodson (1964): Effect of depressive disorders on sleep EEG responses. *Arch Gen Psychiat, 10:*439-445.

INDEX

Freemon, Frank R
    Sleep research: a critical review, by Frank R. Freemon.
Springfield, Ill., Thomas ₍1972₎

    ix, 205 p.   illus.   24 cm. $14.50   **index.**

    Bibliography : p. 161–200.

    1. Sleep—Physiological aspects.   I. Title.

292282 QP425.F74
        ISBN 0-398-02540-1   612'.821   72-75915
                                                                      MARC

        Library of Congress   72 ₍4₎